RESEARCH FOR THE HEALTH PROFESSIONAL

A Practical Guide

RESEARCH FOR THE HEALTH PROFESSIONAL

A Practical Guide

Diana M. Bailey, EdD, OTR
Assistant Professor
Boston School of Occupational Therapy
Tufts University
Medford, Massachusetts

F. A. DAVIS COMPANY • Philadelphia

Printed in the United States of America

Last digit indicates print number: 10 9 8 7 6 5 4 3 2

As new scientific information becomes available through basic and clinical research, recommended treatments and drug therapies undergo changes. The author(s) and publisher have done everything possible to make this book accurate, up to date, and in accord with accepted standards at the time of publication. The authors, editors, and publisher are not responsible for errors or omissions or for consequences from application of the book, and make no warranty, expressed or implied, in regard to the contents of the book. Any practice described in this book should be applied by the reader in accordance with professional standards of care used in regard to the unique circumstances that may apply in each situation. The reader is advised always to check product information (package inserts) for changes and new information regarding dose and contraindications before administering any drug. Caution is especially urged when using new or infrequently ordered drugs.

Library of Congress Cataloging-in-Publication Data

Bailey, Diana M., 1942–
    Research for the health professional : a practical guide / Diana M. Bailey.
        p. cm.
    Includes bibliographical references and index.
    ISBN 0-8036-0554-4 (alk. paper)
    1. Medicine—Research—Methodology.   I. Title.
    [DNLM: 1. Data Collection—methods.   2. Publishing.   3. Research
Design.   4. Writing.   WZ 345 B154r]
    R850.B35   1991
    610′.72—dc20
    DNLM/DLC
    for Library of Congress   91-16168
                                                                              CIP

To Anita who was unendingly patient and understanding when "that darned book" took precedence over pressing life events as well as fun.

FOREWORD

Fear and lack of understanding are by far the two most common barriers facing the beginning researcher. How can we as educators help our students overcome these barriers? This was obviously the question facing Diana Bailey when she decided to write *Research for the Health Professional*.

This book's greatest strength is its unique skill-oriented approach, which helps the reader apply research theory in a practical manner. Numerous worksheets provide incentive to study and learn and a method for testing ideas. Discussion of potential pitfalls and stumbling blocks, and boxed asides of actual occupational and physical therapy literature provide valuable learning tools by illustrating important points clearly and succinctly.

Since occupational and physical therapy practitioners must develop their research skills to substantiate theory and practice and to validate their services, both students and practitioners will find this book extremely helpful in meeting that challenge.

Susan B. O'Sullivan, EdD, PT
Associate Professor
Department of Physical Therapy
University of Lowell
Lowell, Massachusetts

PREFACE

This book is intended for students who are conducting research projects or writing theses and for clinicians who are considering doing research in their clinics. It is not meant to be a comprehensive text on research. Instead it gives a brief and simple overview of the research process, leading the reader in a logical, step-by-step sequence through each stage while providing an opportunity to try out ideas on worksheets at the end of each chapter. For those who have previously taken courses in research and statistics, this book may prove to be a memory-jogger, guiding you through the various steps. Those who have not done research before, and those who are taking their first course in research, will need to use a more detailed text alongside this one.

The manual is designed to be a hands-on working tool containing useful tips on managing potential pitfalls, together with worksheets at each step in the sequence. Readers are expected to move in and out of the process at various points along the way. Although many people enter the research cycle at the question identification stage, some find themselves entering at other points and are comfortable moving backward and forward in no particular sequence. This is possible in the manual because each step is designed as a self-contained unit and can be tackled individually.

The original notion for the book came after I had been asked by working therapists to run workshops to refresh their memories and help them get started on research in their clinics. Typically, these clinicians had completed a thesis or a research project in school and had been working for several years. They were now ready to pursue clinical research but had forgotten some procedures or had lost sight of the larger issues.

Because therapists are usually able to sit down to read professional literature only after a full day's work, this book was kept brief and straightforward, outlining a logical sequence of steps to be followed in designing and implementing a project. Similarly, students studying research for the first time are sometimes apt to lose sight of the greater picture, or even the point of their own projects. The ordering of the information in this book may help them stay on track.

I have included numerous examples from the literature in physical therapy and occupational therapy, which are presented in boxed format. This information was boxed so that if you do not wish to interrupt the flow of the narrative, you may skip the boxes and come back to them later. If you enjoy illustrations sprinkled liberally throughout a text you may prefer to read the boxes as you go along. Often the box gives a brief outline or one small portion of a study in order to make a point; you are encouraged to look up the article in its entirety for a greater understanding of the material.

Because I wanted this book to be utilitarian and pragmatic, I have included a list of stumbling blocks at the end of each chapter. The stumbling blocks include things that are likely to go wrong—and are usually things that have gone wrong for me! The purpose is to give the inexperienced researcher some warning of potential pitfalls so that they may be avoided.

Another feature of the book is the collection of worksheets at the end of each chapter. I have developed these over several years while teaching courses in clinical research and providing workshops for working therapists. I hope you will feel comfortable writing directly on these sheets. If you complete all the worksheets, you will have done much of the work needed for the design and writing of your project. Making the results of the project

ix

known to colleagues via a published article—the ultimate goal for most clinical researchers—will be greatly facilitated if you fill in the worksheets as you go along.

Finally, I hope this workbook will assist and guide you through the research maze and, above all else, that you will enjoy yourself as you go. My aim is to make research enticing and to encourage therapists to give it a try. In Horace's words from *Odes*, Book IV, "He who has begun has half done. Dare to be wise; begin!"

Diana M. Bailey

ACKNOWLEDGMENTS

With heartfelt thanks to:

Sharan Schwartzberg for valuable assistance and for lightening my work load so that this book could be written—and for introducing me to Jean-François;

Jean-François Vilain and Lynn Borders Caldwell for guiding me through the process and making it fun along the way:

The reviewers for their insights and useful suggestions:

Bette Bonder, PhD, OTR/L, FAOTA
Associate Professor and Chair
Department of Health Sciences
Cleveland State University
Cleveland, Ohio

Leonard Elbaum, PT
Associate Professor
Physical Therapy Department
Florida International University
Miami, Florida

Patti Maurer, PhD, OTR
Chair, Department of Occupational
   Therapy
Virginia Commonwealth University
Richmond, Virginia

Terrie Nolinske, MA, OTR, CO,
Assistant Professor
Department of Occupational Therapy
Rush Presbyterian St. Luke's Medical
   Center
Chicago, Illinois

Otto D. Payton, PhD, PT
Director, Graduate Studies
Department of Physical Therapy
Medical College of Virginia
Virginia Commonwealth University
Richmond, Virginia

Louise R. Thibodeaux, MA, OTR/L, FAOTA
Assistant Professor and Director
Graduate Curriculum Development
Division of Occupational Therapy
University of Alabama at Birmingham
Birmingham, Alabama

CONTENTS

ILLUSTRATIONS

TABLES

Introduction

WHAT IS RESEARCH?

Research can be fun, exciting, and fascinating. It is often the case that the student who is required to write a research thesis starts out appalled by the idea yet ends up feeling proud of the results, having enjoyed the challenge. There is a great sense of satisfaction to be derived from completing an exacting, often complex, always stimulating process.

Unfortunately, some people put off attempting research because of preconceived notions. For a few, it conjures up pictures of statistics, rats, and mazes. In fact, research is any activity undertaken to increase our knowledge; it is the systematic investigation of a problem, issue, or question. This may mean reviewing all the literature on a given topic and drawing new conclusions about that topic, or it may mean manipulating certain items to see what happens to other items, or merely searching in an organized manner for existing relationships between characteristics or entities.

Two means of discovering and using knowledge are inductive and deductive reasoning. In using *deductive reasoning*, one accepts or believes a general principle, then applies that principle to the individual case. For example, based on anatomical and physiological information and the resulting theory concerning exercise and joint wear, a therapist may believe that arthritic patients will benefit from receiving short treatment sessions as frequently as possible. Consequently, she will treat the next arthritic patient who is assigned to her caseload 5 days per week for 15- to 20-minute sessions.

In using *inductive reasoning*, one accepts or believes a finding about an individual and then applies that belief to all similar individuals, assuming that it will be true for all. For example, if a therapist finds that a specific arthritic patient benefits more from treatment given five times per week than from treatment given twice per week, she may be inclined to treat all subsequent arthritic patients five times per week.

The problem with deductive reasoning is that although the principle may usually be true, there may well be exceptions. The problem with inductive reasoning is that the individual upon whom you have based the principle may be the exception, so that the principle will probably not then apply to all other cases that follow. This illustrates one inherent problem with the case study approach and points to the reason researchers often try to have as many cases as possible in their research samples, so that they are increasing their chances of developing *real* principles.

RESEARCH IS NOT EASY

Research in the health sciences is not an easy undertaking. Human behavior is extremely complex and, therefore, difficult to isolate and to measure. Because we are working in

1

A. Pure	Applied
Abstract and general, concerned with generating new theory and gaining new knowledge for the knowledge's sake.	Designed to answer a practical question, to help people do their jobs better.
B. Experimental	Descriptive
Manipulating one variable to see its effect on another variable, while controlling for as many other variables as possible and randomly assigning subjects to groups.	Describing a group, a situation, or an individual to gain knowledge which may be applied to further groups or situations, as in case studies or trend analyses.
C. Clinical	Laboratory
Performed in the "real world" where control over variables is quite difficult.	Performed in "unreal" or laboratory surroundings that are tightly controlled.

Figure 1 Description of categories of research.

health fields, there is the added complication that the clients who are the subjects of our research are, by definition, not functioning optimally. Some clients may not want to participate in research studies; there are numerous ethical issues that need to be considered in doing research on human beings. And last, research takes time and other resources that busy clinicians may not have.

CATEGORIZING RESEARCH

There are many ways of labeling and categorizing types of research. For example, research may be pure or applied, experimental or descriptive, clinical or laboratory in nature. Figure 1 describes these three categories.

ESTIMATING TIME FRAMES FOR COMPLETING A RESEARCH PROJECT

Therapists often ask, "How long will it take to complete a research study?" or "How long must I spend at it each day or week?" In my experience advising graduate occupational therapy students in their thesis preparation and writing, it takes them an average of 6 months to 1 year. This includes conceptualizing the issue to be studied, carrying out the project, and writing the study. As students, they are usually not carrying a caseload of clients or tied to a 40-hour work week; however, they do have classes to attend, and often they are working full time on an affiliation.

My experience with research being conducted by therapists in the clinic is that projects tend to take longer—about 1 year to 18 months—with periods of time spent on the project each week. Of course, certain phases of the research demand more or less input. For example, carrying out the actual treatment in a case in which a new treatment approach is being investigated requires that the therapist adhere to the stipulated amount of preparation, treatment, and record keeping, according to the research protocol. Meanwhile, reading the literature or writing the results may be done in one's own time and on a less precise schedule. The therapist working from 9 AM to 5 PM should plan on reading and writing in the evening and on weekends. There are few clinical situations in which therapists are sufficiently free during the day to do the amount of extra work required to complete a research study.

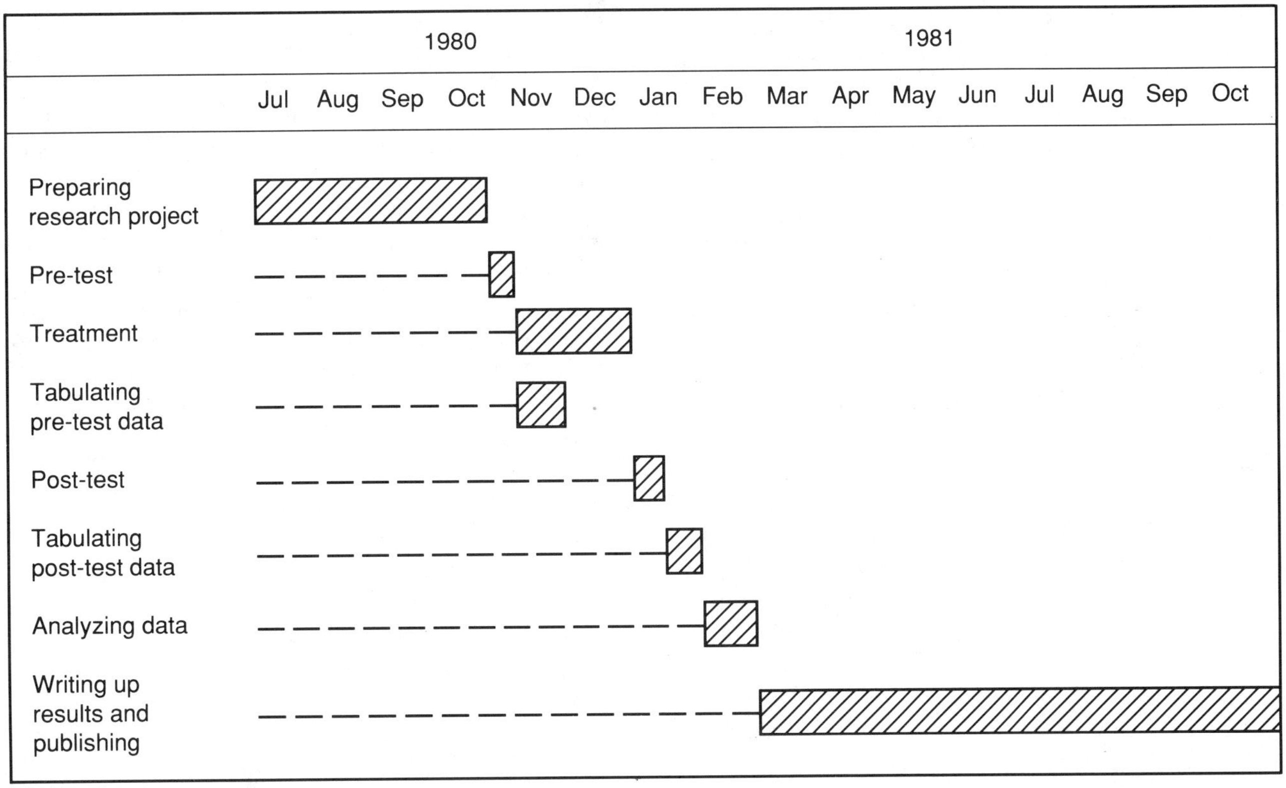

Figure 2 Time chart for conducting a research study.

For example, Figure 2 depicts the amount of time I took to complete a study conducted in a nursing home while I held a full-time teaching position. Changes in speech patterns of chronic schizophrenic patients were investigated following a program of sensory stimulation. The hypothesis was tested using a pre-test and post-test design with an experimental group and a control group.

STEPS IN THE RESEARCH PROCESS

It is useful to remember that research is a circular process. The researcher starts with a question in mind, goes through the investigative stages, and ends up with an answer to the question. More often than not, further questions arise during the analyzing and interpreting of the data, which lead to yet more research ideas.

People often have different points of entry into the research process. Some enjoy starting afresh at the question identification stage, whereas others may happen upon some study results that they question and feel they would like to investigate for themselves. Still others enter at various phases along the way. Whatever the entry point, there is a process or a series of steps that follows a logical sequence:

1. Identifying a problem that needs to be solved or a question that needs to be answered
2. Reviewing the existing writing on that issue
3. Formulating a question or hypothesis about the problem based on the reading
4. Designing a procedure that will address the question or hypothesis
5. Carrying out the procedure
6. Collecting and interpreting the findings
7. Publishing the answer to the question so that others may benefit from the identified knowledge

This book will go through that process step by step, giving the necessary information to understand each step and offering practical hints on how to get over the hurdles that frequently present themselves. There are worksheets at the end of each chapter that can be completed as you read about that step. If you persevere, you will be able to carry out a research project from its inception to publication by working your way through this manual.

The beginning chapters discuss the formulation of a research question or problem, how to review the literature, and how to refine the subject by developing background material and establishing parameters for the study. Next, the decision regarding the research method is examined and various research designs are presented. The section dealing with how to collect and analyze quantitative and qualitative data is followed by a chapter on reporting the results and drawing conclusions from the findings. Finally, how to prepare the study for publication or in thesis format is considered in detail.

CHAPTER

1

Identifying a Question or Problem

WHERE DO RESEARCH TOPICS COME FROM?

Research topics usually come from the work environment. For most therapists, that means the clinic or other patient settings. You may have found you often ask yourself and your co-workers clinically based questions, such as "I wonder why this patient with hemiplegia made more gains than that patient with hemiplegia?"; "What did I do differently, that Mr. Smith complies with his home program but Mr. Brown doesn't?"; "Would a behavioral approach or a sensory integrative approach work better for that group of retarded clients?"; "When I use this particular type of group treatment, there seems to be more response from the patients. I wonder why?"; "Why do we always do it this way? What if we tried . . . ?"

Or you may be reading about other people's treatment programs or ideas that trigger a series of questions in relation to your own treatment. You might see something in other people's findings or recommendations that doesn't agree with your clinical experience. Or you identify gaps in the literature that make it difficult to answer your specific questions (see Box 1–A).

Perhaps you have read a fascinating study that has particular significance for you and decide that you would like to replicate it, either just as it is or with modifications based on your own interests. Replication is an excellent way to learn and to practice the scientific inquiry process (see Boxes 1–B and 1–C).

Clinical practice, the literature, and conference presentations are all legitimate sources

---

Box 1–A
Four physical therapists noticed that "clinical literature *suggests* that lumbar lordosis, pelvic tilt and abdominal muscle function are related to each other." (Emphasis mine.) They further noted that "experimental evidence . . . demonstrating the relationship of abdominal muscle 'strength' . . . , lordosis and pelvic tilt has not been published." This led to their conducting an experimental study to examine if such a relationship really does exist and, in fact, they found "that the three items are not related during normal standing." They conclude: "This study demonstrates the need for re-examination of clinical practice based on assumed relationships. . . ." (Walker, Rothstein, Finncane, & Lamb, 1987; p. 512, 516)

Box 1–B

Middlebrook (1988) replicated a thesis study that had been conducted to see if certain functional movement patterns would elicit a hemodynamic response. The original study was conducted on college students who were in the 18- to 22-years age range. Middlebrook was interested to see whether similar findings would exist in an older population and replicated the study using subjects in the 60- to 80-years age range.

---

for research topics. However, there are some things to keep in mind when deciding upon a topic:

- Choose an area of study that fascinates you. Research is a lengthy, sometimes tedious business with many pitfalls. If you aren't excited about your topic to begin with, you most certainly won't be by the time you finish. If you should lose the drive to find the answer to your question, it is almost guaranteed that you won't finish the study.
- Keep it simple. It is very tempting to add on some "juicy" subquestions to see whether those can be answered at the same time. However, this may result in your not knowing which variables are responsible for which changes. It is generally better to try to answer one question at a time.
- Do a pilot study to iron out the "kinks" before starting the main study. A pilot study is a smaller version of the main study and will allow you to see if there are any problems in the design. (Pilot studies are described in Chapter 9.) Such a study can save innumerable headaches later and prevent the feeling that you would have done a whole host of things differently had you known then what you know now.
- Keep writing things down to clarify your thinking—the question, variables, definitions, methods. Whenever you have a brainstorm about your project, take a minute to write it down.

Ending up with a researchable question is undoubtedly a difficult task, and people go about it in different ways. However most people go through several common stages, including having an idea, thinking about the idea, discussing the idea with colleagues to see if it makes sense, checking in the literature to see if it makes sense, deciding exactly what goals are to be achieved through the research, and, finally, defining the questions more precisely to formulate the hypotheses.

IDENTIFYING A REASONABLE QUESTION

This may well be the most difficult step in the research process. First of all, what makes a question reasonable? By *reasonable* we mean that the study will be related to one's profession, will serve some useful purpose, will add to the profession's body of knowledge,

---

Box 1–C

In *Two Approaches to Improving the Functional Performance of a Head-Injured Adult*, the efficacy of two occupational therapy approaches—functional and transfer of training—was examined. Rabideau's study (1985) examined which of the two treatment approaches is more effective in rehabilitating functional performance of cognitively impaired head-injured adults. In 1989, Loftus replicated the study, holding all variables constant except for the cognitive level of functioning of the subjects. She hypothesized that the results would be different based on her clinical experience with head-injured adults, hence Loftus was changing a variable in a study because her knowledge and experience told her that the study results would change if the degree of symptoms in the subjects was different.

Box 1-D

Parker and Chan (1986) studied stereotyping among occupational and physical therapists because they felt that their study would have importance in those therapists' ability or inability to work together effectively as members of a team.

and will be "do-able." This means it will be possible to convert it into a research design, there will be an instrument to measure the variables, and the subjects and other resources needed will be available. To be reasonable and researchable a question must have the following attributes:

- A rationale or *theory base*. How will this study add to the body of knowledge of the profession? Does it fall into an existing treatment approach (e.g., developmental, behavioral, biomechanical, rehabilitative) so that it will add to the theoretical base of the approach? The project is more useful to clinicians if it is based on a theory with which they are familiar and through which they can refine their treatment.
- There must be *significance* to your question. Who cares whether or not you answer this question? Will you be proud of the contribution of knowledge you have made to your profession? This is the *so what* of the study. When you describe your study to someone and he or she asks, "So what?" can you give that person a good answer (see Boxes 1-D and 1-E)? Try to think about possible outcomes of your study to be sure that your work will be worthwhile. Although experienced researchers sometimes engage in research that is of a philosophical bent where the benefit is not immediately apparent, it is better for the beginning researcher to engage in studies in which there are clear implications that either the clients or the program will benefit as a result (see Box 1-F).
- What variables will you be studying? A *variable* is any attribute or characteristic that can vary, such as diagnosis, age, heart rate, elbow flexion, and self-esteem. Can your variables be identified and measured? Some variables are easy to identify—particularly visual ones such as height, eye color, or grip strength as measured on a dynamometer—but others—such as non-verbal communication, professionalism, and schizophrenia—are more difficult to identify and to characterize. Some variables are straightforward to measure (e.g., joint angles, weight, heart rate), whereas others require complicated measuring instruments (e.g., job satisfaction, sense of mastery, altruism, dysphasia).

Variables may be expected to change and to be measured in some studies but may be held constant, or unchanging, in others. The *same* variable may be changeable in one study but held constant in another. For example, task attention may be measured in 9-, 10-, 11-, and 12-year-olds, whereas in a different study, a group of 12-year-olds may be tested for a relationship between reading comprehension and level of attention. Age would be a changing variable in the first study and would be held constant in the second.

Many studies look for relationships between variables (Is this variable related to that one? If so, how?). Other studies, however, look for a cause-and-effect relation-

Box 1-E

Physical therapists compared the reliability and validity of four instruments that have been used for a similar purpose: to measure lumbar spine and pelvic positions (Burdett, Brown, & Fall, 1986). They felt it would be useful to know if one instrument was more reliable and appropriate than the others so that therapists could select the best tool. If there was no difference, then such issues as expense, ease of use, and convenience for patients could be considered in selecting an instrument.

Box 1–F

In a survey following a therapeutic work program for head-injured adults (Lyons & Morse, 1988), it was found that a greater percentage of clients than that reported by other prevocational programs were participating in occupational activities at follow-up. The activities, counseling, scheduling, and other components of the vocational program under study were clearly of benefit to head-injured clients.

---

ship between variables (If this variable is changed, does it have an effect on that one? If so, what effect?). For example, Nelson (1989) was trying to determine whether there was a relationship between therapists' professionalism and their self-esteem. She was conducting *correlational research*. Middlebrook (1988) wanted to see if certain functional movement patterns had an effect on hemodynamic responses in older individuals. She was engaging in *experimental research*. Different types of research designs are explained in Chapter 5.

- What *resources*—such as money, time, computer use, and statistical assistance— will you need to carry out the project, and are those resources available to you? Does the question you have in mind require extensive statistical analysis to find the answer? If so and you do not have the services of a statistician at hand, is this a reasonable project for you?
- What *subjects* will you need to carry out the project, and are those subjects available to you? It is invariably more practical for clinicians to include in their studies patients or clients at their own facility rather than to try to locate certain types of patients, such as those with a specific diagnosis, who may be found only at other facilities. Using patients you can easily reach greatly increases the chance of the project being completed.

THE PURPOSE OF THE STUDY

Setting the specific research aims and objectives for your research is most important and should be done early in the process. It is accomplished by establishing a hypothesis. What is it you want to achieve for your clients, your program, or the profession as a result of your project (see Box 1–G)?

What do you think might be changed for the better, according to your results? Stout (1988), for example, thinks that occupational therapists have the skills and knowledge to be involved in planning children's playgrounds and that if they participate in this activity, more playgrounds will be accessible and available for children with disabilities.

Box 1–G

In a multicase study described in the *American Journal of Occupational Therapy* (Giles & Clark-Wilson, 1988), the purpose was to improve the washing and dressing skills of four adults with brain injury. All were heavily dependent on others in their personal hygiene. The authors were investigating the benefits of a specific treatment approach that they hoped would assist other patients with their washing and dressing skills.

THE HYPOTHESIS

What is your hunch about the possible outcome of your research? The answer to this question will help you formulate the hypothesis. The hypothesis may or may not be supported at the end of the research, but it is important to postulate what may happen. The purpose of the hypothesis is to suggest new experiments, and new ways of looking at clinical practice, and it is the tool that is used to guide the research process. Some examples of hypotheses from the occupational and physical therapy literature follow.

- There is no significant correlation between grip strength and hand function in the normal population.
- Dominant hands will have a different pattern of correlation between strength and function than non-dominant hands.
- Guided visual imagery will be effective in treating patients with psychosomatic, psychogenic, or chronic somatic disorders.
- The Trager Psychophysical Integration Method will improve the chest mobility of patients with chronic lung disease.
- Prior knowledge will influence the automatic and voluntary postural adjustments of healthy and hemiplegic subjects.
- Age will influence prosthesis use in subjects with above-knee amputation.
- There is a positive relationship between the self-esteem of female occupational therapists and their attitudes/behaviors toward professionalism.
- Occupational health promotion is a viable practice area for occupational therapists.
- Chronic psychiatric patients will live out unsatisfying patterns of maladaptive behavior characterized by:

    Poor balance of work, leisure, activities of daily living, and sleep
    Poor planning for the future reflected in use of time
    Dissatisfaction regarding use of time.

As you can see, the hypothesis is the essence of a research study. All the variables that will be studied are mentioned, together with the expected effect of the interrelationships of those variables. Formulating hypotheses will be discussed in more detail in Chapter 3.

STUMBLING BLOCKS

When problems in carrying out your research begin to look insurmountable and to overwhelm you, having a colleague work with you on the project can be an enormous help. My guess is that far more studies are completed that have two or more researchers than those that have one. When the inevitable problems get one person down, there is someone else who still has some energy to deal with them, so the project can move forward. Perhaps the first person will have the time and inclination to fight the battles next time. Although it is heartily recommended that you work with a colleague, it may make finding a question that interests both of you and meets all the criteria more difficult.

Talking with others about your ideas for a research topic is an excellent idea, but it can prevent you from actually getting started. Everyone has his or her own pet theory about how the project should be carried out, what variables should be measured, and which book should be read to enlighten one on the topic. Listening to and acting upon some of these ideas can be most helpful in shaping your research but also will present conflicting opinions, which must be reconciled somehow. There comes a time when you must decide you have had enough input from colleagues, family, and friends. At this point, the project must be designed and you must "go with it," or you will never get started. This does not mean that you cannot make minor changes as you go along if compelling reasons arise. However, too much advice can be confusing and overwhelming and sometimes can bog the researchers down so that the project never gets started.

WORKSHEETS

Jot down questions that have been in your mind from your clinical practice or discussions with your colleagues. Choose questions about which you are very curious and to which you would love to know the answer.

Look over your list, and decide which question interests you the most. Rank your questions in order of fascination.

Write the number one question here:

Answer these questions about your chosen topic:

Why does it excite you?

Do you *really* want to know the answer?

Is it a simple question or does it have several parts?

Is it possible to do a pilot study on this question to see if it is feasible?

Is there an obvious theory base for this question? If so, name it here:

In your opinion, does this question address a significant problem? If so, answer the question "So what?" here:

What variables will you be studying? List them here:

At first glance, does it appear to you that you will be able to find a way to identify and to measure those variables?

Take a guess at the resources you might need to study this question:

Time

Money

Equipment

Computer

Statistician

Fellow therapists

Other

What type of subjects will you need to study this question?

Are these people available?

Repeat this investigation process for your second identified question, and so on, until you find the most favorable. Remember that your question must be reasonable and researchable.

If you encounter what appear to be insoluble problems with each question, don't despair. This is probably because you are not yet familiar with the variety of methodological options available to you in the research process. Read on, and in subsequent chapters you may find methods you can use that will solve some of these problems.

REFERENCES

Burdett, R.G., Brown, K.E., & Fall, M.P. (1986). Reliability and validity of four instruments for measuring lumbar spine and pelvic positions. *Physical Therapy, 66*(5), 677–684.

Giles, M.G., & Clark-Wilson, J. (1988). The use of behavioral techniques in functional skills training after severe brain injury. *American Journal of Occupational Therapy, 42*(10), 658–665.

Loftus, S.K. (1989). *Two approaches to improving functional performance of a head injured adult: A replication.* Unpublished master's thesis, Tufts University, Medford, MA.

Lyons, J.L., & Morse, A.R. (1988). A therapeutic work program for head-injured adults. *American Journal of Occupational Therapy, 42*(6), 364–370.

Middlebrook, J.A. (1988). *The effect of functional movement patterns on hemodynamic responses in older individuals.* Unpublished master's thesis, Tufts University, Medford, MA.

Nelson, B.J. (1989). *Self-esteem and professionalism in female occupational therapists.* Unpublished master's thesis, Tufts University, Medford, MA.

Parker, H.J., & Chan, F. (1986). Stereotyping: Physical and occupational therapists characterize themselves and each other. *Physical Therapy, 66*(5), 668–672.

Rabideau, G. (1985). *Two approaches to improving the functional performance of a head injured adult.* Unpublished master's thesis, Tufts University, Medford, MA.

Stout, J. (1988). Planning playgrounds for children with disabilities. *American Journal of Occupational Therapy, 42*(10), 653–657.

Walker, M.L., Rothstein, J.M., Finncane, S.D., & Lamb, R.L. (1987). Relationship between lumbar lordosis, pelvic tilt, and abdominal muscle performance. *Physical Therapy, 67*(4), 512–516.

ADDITIONAL READING

Berger, R.M., & Patchner, M.A. (1988). *Planning for research: A guide for the helping professions.* No. 50 in the Sage Human Services Guide Series. Newbury Park, CA: Sage Publications.

Boer, M.R., & Gall, M.D. (1973). Selecting and defining a research problem. In Hubbard, A.W. (Ed.): *Research methods in health, physical education, and recreation.* Washington, DC: American Association of Health and Physical Education Research.

Ethridge, D., & McSweeney, M. (1970). Research in occupational therapy. Part I Introduction. *American Journal of Occupational Therapy, XXIV*(7), 490–493.

Ethridge, D., & McSweeney, M. (1970). Research in occupational therapy. Part II The hypothesis. *American Journal of Occupational Therapy, XXIV*(8), 551–555.

Lehmkuhl, D. (1970). Let's reduce the understanding gap. Part I The question: What and why? *Physical Therapy, 50*, 61–65.

McLaren, H.M. (1973). So you want to conduct a clinical study. *Physiotherapy Canada, 25*, 219–224.

Reviewing the Literature

Now that you have explored some research questions and found one that you would like to answer, the next step is to review what has been written on your topic. Many novice researchers ask, "Why is this necessary? Why can't I just start in on my project?" There are several reasons:

1. Perhaps someone has already researched your question, or one just like it, and the answer is already published. You certainly would not want to waste your time and that of your subjects by repeating what has already been accomplished.
2. Perhaps someone has tried to investigate your question or one very similar and met with insurmountable problems (e.g., not finding a test instrument sensitive enough to measure one of the crucial variables or not being able to control enough of the intervening variables to have confidence in the results). This information would be useful before embarking on a similar project.
3. Perhaps someone has researched your question or one very similar but not in the same way that you intend to research it. You may plan to use slightly different methods or subject characteristics. You would, however, want to benefit from the information that could be gleaned from the previous study.
4. Someone may have already studied one component of the topic and you can build on his or her research, saving yourself time and energy.
5. You will wish to place your study in context with similar studies, so that the reader will know how to perceive your work.
6. It is a good idea to place the study within the theoretical base in which the topic falls (e.g., biomechanical or behavioral theory), again for the reader's benefit, as well as for your increased understanding of the topic.
7. It will be reassuring to find reasons in the literature to suggest why the study you propose will address the problem and how your study is capable of solving the problem or answering the question.
8. It is probable that while searching the literature evidence will be found that will prompt you to change your question. It may need a different emphasis; you may decide to look for a correlational effect rather than a cause and effect; you may refine the sample; and so on.
9. There are strongly held impressions in any profession about various areas of practice—things with which most clinicians would agree. However, impressions are not good enough as the basis for research, and documentation of these beliefs through the literature is always needed (see Walker, Rothstein, Finncane, & Lamb, 1987, cited in Box 1–A).

So, it can be seen that a thorough review of written material on the proposed topic of study is essential if the researcher is to design a relevant, original, helpful, and timely research study.

Box 2-A

In studying the temporal adaptation of chronic psychiatric patients, therapists reviewed literature in the areas of use of time in the "normal" population and in the chronic psychiatric population, the human drive to explore and to master the environment, purposeful activity and the productive use of time, the environment and demographics of people similar to those in the sample, and methods of measuring temporal adaptation.

Box 2-B

Another example would be the study of the effect of technological aids on the exploration behavior of mentally retarded adults. This study necessitated exploring the range of such available aids, other populations using technological devices to improve exploration behavior, as well as an overview of the literature on exploration behavior per se.

In addition to articles and books that pertain strictly to your chosen subject, it is important to read related material so that you are well versed in the whole topic being studied. Some examples of such reading are given in Boxes 2-A, 2-B, and 2-C. From these examples, it may be seen that breadth of reading is as important as depth of reading in order to prepare an effective research proposal.

HOW TO GO ABOUT A LITERATURE SEARCH

You will likely find material relevant to your topic in journals, books, and government documents. Because much of the material relevant to occupational and physical therapy will be found in the medical, social, educational, anthropological, psychological and engineering sciences, the best place to locate material is in institutional libraries, such as those found in universities, postgraduate medical centers, training institutions for health care professionals, and other institutions of higher learning. Although this may cause problems for the clinician who is isolated geographically, frequently material can be found through the public library through use of interlibrary loan. However, this service may require a wait of several weeks before the receipt of material.

Once a well-stocked library and a helpful librarian have been located, it is necessary to decide whether you will do a hand search or a computer search of the literature. For a hand search, the following will be used:

1. The card catalog (now often computerized) and reference books to find relevant books on your topic
2. US government documents for relevant government writings
3. The indexes and abstracts to find relevant articles in journals

THE CARD CATALOG AND REFERENCE BOOKS

There is a card in the library catalog for every item housed in the library, except for individual journal articles. There are three cards for every item, filed by author's last name, by title, and by subject. If the system has been computerized, there will be equivalent entries in the computer data base for author's name, title, and subject. If you are aware of leading authorities in your topic area—such as A. Jean Ayres in the area of sensory integrative techniques, or Signe Brunnstrom in kinesiology—you can look up in the catalog, or call up on the computer, those authors' names and review titles to find appropriate

Box 2-C

For a study in *Physical Therapy* regarding prosthetic use by elderly patients with dysvascular above-knee and through-knee amputations (Beckman & Axtell, 1987), the literature survey included statistics on the whole population, followed by those on the elderly population who are undergoing amputations; conditions commonly leading to amputations; review of the literature concerning whether or not to fit the elderly amputee patient with a prosthesis, including such topics as costs versus benefits, physical limitations, motivation, training time, and the likelihood of the patient using the prosthesis upon discharge; and finally, an overview of studies describing functional outcomes of prosthetic use by elderly people. Additionally, the authors stated that they had limited their literature search to the past 15 years because of recent changes in surgical procedures and rehabilitation care and improvements in prostheses.

books. If you are not aware of experts in the field, the subject index/data base should be used to find appropriate books or journals. Unfortunately, searching for books by subject can be somewhat frustrating if you are not aware of how the subject terms are chosen. An important point to keep in mind is that the catalog makes use of a specialized vocabulary, sometimes quite unlike the terms used in everyday language. Here are some examples:

Everyday language	*Catalog language*
films; movies	moving pictures
abstract art	art, abstract
Vietnam war	Vietnamese conflict

In the catalog, however, there are often guide cards or prompts in the computer program that refer the researcher to the correct subject heading. There is also a two-volume list of Library of Congress subject headings, usually kept near the catalog, to assist one in finding the right words for a topic.

There are several reference books that might be helpful for investigating a topic in general rather than something specific to a health field. *Books in Print* and *British Books in Print* are huge tomes containing every book currently available. Each consists of four separate volumes, one each for authors, subjects, titles, and publishers. Incidentally, the 1987 to 1988 *Books in Print* has occupational therapy listed as a subject and contains 93 entries. Physical therapy lists 104 entries. Other useful reference books are the *Annual Reviews* which are published in specific content areas and which exist in such fields as psychology and physiology.

US GOVERNMENT DOCUMENTS

Select libraries around the country are depositories for US government publications. This collection is arranged by the Superintendent of Documents' classification scheme and is updated monthly. It lists publications issued by all branches of the US government, including congressional, department, and bureau publications. Issues are indexed in separate volumes for authors, titles/key words, subjects, and series or report titles. The type of documents likely to be useful to therapists include amendments to the Medicare law, Public Law 94-142 Equal Educational Opportunities, the Report of the President's Commission on Mental Health, and the law concerning the disabled and architectural barriers.

JOURNAL INDEXES AND ABSTRACTS

A hand search of the journal indexes and abstracts requires that the subject terms be isolated unless the authors of specific articles are known. The volumes are organized by subject and sometimes by author and are often bound 1 year at a time. It is necessary to define the subject being researched carefully in order to locate relevant articles because terminology can be peculiar to the field and can vary from field to field (e.g., one index may use the term *adolescent* whereas another uses *teenager*). The following are the most useful indexes for therapists:

1. *Index Medicus*, which contains entries from the major medically related journals around the world (approximately 4680 of them) and which is updated monthly. Entries from the *American Journal of Occupational Therapy* and *Physical Therapy* are included in the *Complete Index Medicus*. However, the *American Journal of Occupational Therapy* is not included in the *Abridged Index Medicus*, so be sure to specify to the librarian which version you want. There is an accompanying volume of *Medical Subject Headings* to assist in locating subject terms, together with the codes for computer searching of the *Index Medicus*.

2. Professional journals of the major health fields also have their own indexes. The *American Journal of Occupational Therapy* is indexed by subject and author and is cumulative from 1972 to 1983 and annual thereafter. *Physical Therapy* is also indexed by subject and author on an annual basis. These indexes are generally available only in the libraries of universities with training programs in those specific professions.

3. Three other indexes likely to be helpful for therapists are the *Resources in Education* (RIE), the *Current Index to Journals in Education* (CIJE), and the more recent *Exceptional Child Educational Resource* (ECER). The RIE abstracts educational research reports by subject, author, and institution, and most reports are available on microfilm. The CIJE and ECER abstract articles in education and education-related journals by subject, author, and journal content. They are companions to RIE, and all three form the content for the computer data base of the Educational Resources Information Center (ERIC). There is an accompanying thesaurus of ERIC terms.

4. *Psychological Abstracts* is an index that contains abstracts of books, journal articles, technical reports, and scientific documents concerning psychology. It uses a classified arrangement with author and subject indexes and has cumulative indexes by year. There is a thesaurus of psychological index terms as a companion volume. Figure 2–1 shows an example of what would be found in looking up the entry for *cognitive ability*. The major terms used for *cognitive ability* in the indexes are *cognitive functioning* and *intellectual functioning*, but the narrower terms *mathematical, reading, spatial,* and *verbal ability* also are found in the index. The book suggests that the reader may be

```
Cognitive Ability                          73

PN 1504          SC 10050

SN Level of functioning in intellectual tasks
   UF   Cognitive Functioning
        Intellectual Functioning
   N    Mathematical Ability           73
        Reading Ability                73
        Spatial Ability                82
        Verbal Ability                 67
   R    Ability                        67


Key: PN  —  Postings Note
     SN  —  Scope notes available
     UF  —  Used for term
     N   —  Narrower term
     R   —  Related term
```

Figure 2–1 Thesaurus entry for the term *cognitive ability* in the Psychological Abstracts.

interested in the related term *ability*. The numbers are used for entering these terms on the computer, should one be doing a computer search.

5. *Sociological Abstracts* includes abstracts from some sociology books and from sociological and social science journals in various languages. There is a classified arrangement of abstracts with access by subject terms; however, some feel that the subject headings are poorly defined and thus find this index difficult to use.

6. *Dissertation Abstracts* can be another useful source of research studies and also can be hand searched. One problem with using dissertations as reference material is that if you come across a study that is relevant to your project and decide that you would like to review the study in its entirety, you must either send away for a paper copy of the dissertation—which may cost from $20 to $35—or find a library that has microfilm copies of dissertations. However, the *Dissertation Abstracts* volumes themselves contain comprehensive abstracts of the studies, which may be sufficient for your purposes. The volumes are divided into two major categories: sciences/engineering and humanities/social sciences. Other indexes and abstracts useful for therapists are listed in Appendix A.

Most indexes and abstracts are bound 1 year at a time, so it is necessary to look through several volumes of the same index, depending on how far back in time you wish to search. How far back to look is something for careful consideration. If the subject is rapidly developing and a great deal is currently being written about it (e.g., acquired immune deficiency syndrome, or the plight of the homeless, or Alzheimer's disease), then 2 to 5 years may be sufficient to give you volumes of material on the most up-to-date thinking. If the subject has been developed over many years (topics such as personal values or carpal tunnel syndrome) and has remained fairly stable in content since the original work, it may be wise to go back to the time of most plentiful writing on that topic in order to find the classic works—sometimes as many as 20 or 30 years. If one or two articles or books are constantly referred to in more recent works, those are probably the classic and important writings related to that topic. It would be well to read those for a more thorough grasp of the topic.

COMPUTER SEARCHES

For speed and thoroughness, you may decide to conduct a computer search of the literature, requiring a facility that has that capability. Most university libraries have access to on-line computer searches of journal indexes. MEDLINE is the data base associated with *Index Medicus* and provides access to more than half a million entries, recognizing some 13,000 subject headings. ERIC is the data base formulated from the RIE, CIJE, and ECER, and PsycINFO comes from the *Psychological Abstracts* and uses a content classification scheme that divides the field of psychology into 16 major categories and 64 subcategories.

Often, a librarian will perform the hands-on search, but you must do the preparation. This entails having the research question well thought out and having the terms (sometimes called *descriptors* or *key words*) identified. The terms come from the thesaurus that accompanies each index (Box 2–D).

Box 2–D

In a study on therapist attrition from occupational therapy (Bailey, 1990), terms were identified by the researcher as *employee turnover*; *personnel turnover*; *career mobility*; *job involvement*; *career change*; *tenure*; and *occupational aspirations*. These terms were found in the thesauruses accompanying the *Index Medicus* and the *Psychological Abstracts*. As mentioned previously, different indexes and abstracts use different terms to identify similar subjects. Thus, one index used the term *employee turnover*, whereas another used *personnel turnover*.

Box 2-E

The above search on attrition was conducted on the MEDLINE, PsycINFO, and ERIC data bases. The MEDLINE search actually took 5 minutes on line and cost $3.75. Using the terms *occupational* and *physical therapists, social workers, personnel turnover*, and *career mobility*, 84 titles were generated, of which 10 looked relevant and were printed with abstracts. Of these 10 articles, 3 were located, and 1 was eventually used in the publication. In the PsycINFO search on the same topic, the terms *occupational, physical, and speech therapists*; *social workers*; *psychologists*; *nurses*; *mobility*; *tenure*; *employee turnover*; *career change*; and *job involvement* were used. The search took 5.25 minutes on line, cost $5.58, and generated 82 titles. Nineteen of those titles appeared relevant and were abstracted. Of these, 15 were located, and 5 were actually used in the article. In the ERIC search, the terms *occupational, physical*, and *speech therapists*; *social workers*; *nurses*; *turnover*; *career change*; and *occupational mobility* were used to generate 57 titles. The relevant 15 were abstracted, 7 were located, and 4 were eventually used. This search took 2.5 minutes on line and cost $3.02. Preparation for the search, including finding useful terms in the thesauruses, took about 30 minutes.

If you cannot find the topic under one heading, try another. It is quicker to look through the list of terms in the accompanying thesaurus than to wrack your brain for possible alternative words. It is preferable to sit with the librarian while he or she is on line with the computer, so that you can make decisions if changes need to be made in term selection.

There is quite a range of costs for computer searches, depending on the data base used and the facility where the search is performed. Sometimes there is a special price offer for use of specific data bases during a given week, which will cut the cost dramatically (see Boxes 2-E and 2-F).

Selecting the data base to be searched (e.g., MEDLINE or ERIC) will depend on which field you think will contain material relevant to your project, such as medicine, sociology, or education. Once the terms are entered, the computer will scan all the material in that data base for articles keyed in with those words for as far back as you wish. Terms can be *crossed* with one another, so that you receive only those articles keyed in with both terms, for example, *arthritis* and *joint protection*. You can ask for three or four terms to be listed for each article but are likely to get very few responses if you are this specific. It is often cost effective to have only titles printed out at first, so that the items that appear most promising can be selected before asking for an abstract. You will be paying for the amount of time the computer is actually on line, that is, searching and producing material. Thus, it is well to be prepared ahead and not to be thinking out terms and alternative strategies while logged on to the computer.

LOCATING ARTICLES AND BOOKS

Once a list of articles and books has been obtained from the computer search, the titles and/or abstracts must be reviewed to see if they appear relevant to the study. You must then go to the book stacks, the periodical room, or the government documents depository to

---

Box 2-F

A search on schizophrenic patients' use of time cost $32 in total and yielded 204 titles, 27 of which were actually related to the topic. This search was conducted on MEDLINE and PsycINFO and took 8 minutes logged on to the computer. A search on the same topic in the *Mental Health Abstracts* produced six articles, only one of which was relevant, for a cost of $2.40. A final search of this subject in the *Sociological Abstracts* cost $6.70, produced an additional eight articles, of which two were useful. Preparation for the search on schizophrenic patients' use of time was about 1 hour, because this was a difficult subject to pin down.

find the items. You will be expected to locate books and journal articles on your own with the aid of the number from the catalog card/computer data base and a map of the library showing where groups of numbers are located. Periodical rooms are usually organized alphabetically according to the title of the periodical. However, one must usually ask for assistance in a government documents depository, and the librarian will bring the item to you.

If an article is only peripherally related to your topic, you can jot down the relevant points together with the complete reference while you are in the library. However, it will probably be preferable to make copies of the most pertinent articles or to check out the most relevant books so that it is possible to study them at your leisure.

ORGANIZING THE MATERIAL

You have doubtless heard of the infamous index cards in reference to organizing literature searches. They are an extremely useful way of keeping information so that it is manageable and retrievable. Many people find the 5″ × 8″ size to be most useful. Take a package to the library and jot down information from the peripheral articles and books directly on the cards — a separate card per article or book. Cards on the more important or complicated articles of which you made copies can be completed at your convenience at home. Arrange the information in the same way on each card. Figures 2–2 and 2–3 illustrate how cards may be completed.

At the top of the card, it is helpful to add the more specific subject area within the general research topic, such as those mentioned in Box 2–G. Cards can then be grouped by subject areas, which will make writing up the material easier. When more than one subject area is mentioned in an article or book, it is possible to cross-reference and to have a card in each section for that article or book. At the end of the most useful articles — ones that are most relevant to the topic — be sure to peruse the reference lists. These can be a most useful source of additional reading.

As soon as you have read and prepared cards on all the articles and books, you are ready to write the review. Start by reviewing the subject headings at the top of the index cards and putting them in a logical sequence (see Box 2–H). In this way, the reader is carried through a progression of topics pertinent to the study. By the end of the literature review, the reader should understand why the project was being undertaken.

Decision to fit the elderly with prostheses
Beckman, C.E. & Axtell, L.A.
Prosthetic use in elderly patients with
dysvascular above-knee and through-knee
amputations.
Physical Therapy, 67(10), 1510-1516   1987
Contains a thorough review of literature on
whether or not to fit the elderly with prostheses.
Includes:
    costs versus benefits
    physical limitations
    motivation
    training time
    likelihood of patient using prosthesis.
Plus, an overview of studies describing functional
outcomes of prosthetic use by elderly.

Figure 2-2 Sample card completed for an article.

Berger, R.M. & Patchner, M.A.
Planning for research: A guide for the helping
professions.
#50 in Sage Human Services Guide Series.
Newbury Park, CA: Sage Publications   1988
A comprehensive description of the planning
stages for a research project:
    finding the question
    stating the purpose
    stating the significance
    deciding on the design.

Figure 2-3 Sample card completed for a book.

Next, concentrate on one group of cards at a time. Look for common themes that run through the various authors' papers and make a note of the themes on a separate card. If a sole author makes a point you would like to include, mark it. Now look at these themes and important points. Do they fall in a logical sequence? Do they flow from one to the other, making the progression of ideas you want to convey to the reader? Write these ideas down in sequence and see if there are steps left out. If so, add them in your own words. When you are satisfied that you have stated the important issues about this topic in a clear, concise manner, add the authors' names whose ideas you have cited, together with the year of publication, in parentheses after each idea. You are now ready to move on to the next major subject area of your literature review and to repeat the process.

It is a real challenge to write a literature review well. Try to avoid starting every sentence with "Smith (1988) says . . ." or "Brown (1989) feels that. . . ." Read through some literature sections in published articles to get some ideas for imaginative ways to start sentences and ways to incorporate several authors' ideas and findings in one or two sentences. There are space constraints in journals, so you will not be able to devote many paragraphs to the literature summary. In fact, you will probably read many more articles and books than you will be able to include. Restrict yourself to the most important and convincing work on the points you wish to make. Refer to the articles listed in Appendix B for well-written literature reviews.

The format used to cite references is most specific, and each journal has a required format. Styles will be addressed in detail in Chapter 11 of this book in the section on publishing an article.

HOW LONG SHOULD THE LITERATURE REVIEW BE?

The length of a literature review varies greatly depending on the type of document being produced. For the student writing a thesis, the literature review should be comprehensive and should demonstrate that all literature relevant to the study has been examined and

Box 2-G

If a researcher were trying to identify factors related to prosthetic candidacy in elderly people, likely subject headings might include "Types of prostheses," "Incidence and causes of amputation in elderly people," "Decision to fit the elderly patient with prostheses," "Physical limitations and motivation factors," "Costs versus benefits," "Training procedures," and "Functional outcomes."

Box 2–H

If you were writing the review of the study concerning prostheses mentioned earlier, it would be logical to order the subjects in the following way:

1. Causes and incidence of amputation in elderly people
2. Types of prostheses
3. Decision to fit the elderly patient with prostheses
4. Costs versus benefits
5. Physical limitations and motivation
6. Training procedures
7. Functional outcomes

that the most important material has been analyzed. All literature should be examined that explains the problem, suggests why your study is appropriate to it, describes your study's capability for solving the problem, and relates to any other studies that have attempted to solve the problem. Consequently, a thesis literature review may typically run from 20 to 40 pages.

The literature review for a journal article, on the other hand, tends to be brief and to the point. This is because there are space constraints imposed by journal editors, and there is often a requirement that an entire article be kept to within five to seven printed pages. The *Publication Manual of the American Psychological Association* (1983) offers helpful guidelines for what to include in the background or literature review section of a journal article (see Box 2–I).

Completing the literature review is a major step in the right direction. It does not have to be written in final form at this stage of the project, of course, but it is certainly a potential hurdle, and it is a good idea to get the writing accomplished as soon as possible. You are now ready to refine your research question and to develop the background material for your study, based on what you have read.

STUMBLING BLOCKS

By including *all* the reference information immediately on the index cards, you will save yourself time and trouble when you are ready to prepare the reference list. This is the moment when it is common to find that you have:

- lost the article
- returned the book
- loaned the article to someone else
- spilled coffee on the volume number.

A common problem is arriving at the library, finding just the articles you have been looking for, and not having enough change to make the copies. It is wise to take a roll of dimes to the library with you for copying purposes. In some libraries, you may purchase a plastic credit card that can be inserted in the copying machine and is good for the number of copies that you paid for in advance. Most libraries have one or more copying machines outside their periodical rooms and expect patrons to make copies of journal articles. Bound journals may not be taken out of the library, whereas all books except reference books may be checked out.

While immersed in piles of journals or computer printouts, it is common to lose sight of the topics being sought and to get sidetracked into other interesting areas. I find it helpful to have in front of me a card containing my research question and a list of the major areas

---

Box 2-1

"Discuss the literature but do not include an exhaustive historical review. Assume that the reader has knowledge in the field for which you are writing and does not require a complete digest. Although you should acknowledge the contributions of others to the study of the problem, cite only that research pertinent to the specific issue and avoid references with only tangential or general significance. If you summarize earlier works, avoid nonessential details; instead, emphasize pertinent findings, relevant methodological issues, and major conclusions. Refer the reader to general surveys or reviews of the topic if they are available.

"Demonstrate the logical continuity between previous and present work. Develop the problem with enough breadth and clarity to make it generally understood by as wide a professional audience as possible. Do not let the goal of brevity mislead you into writing a statement intelligible only to the specialist."

(American Psychological Association, 1983, p. 25)

---

for which I am searching, as illustrated in Figure 2-4. When I feel as if I may be straying too far afield or have forgotten the major issues, I glance at this card and it gets me back on track.

If during a computer search you cannot find any sources or very few sources relevant to your topic, there are several possibilities of what may be happening:

1. Your topic does not make sense. No one has written in this area because it is not logical and there is nothing there to research.
2. You are looking in the wrong data base (e.g., you are looking in medicine and should be in vocational services).
3. You have virgin territory; nothing has been done in your area. That is very exciting—go ahead!

Because many people find writing literature reviews a tiresome task—one that they put off as long as possible—promptness is definitely the best policy, and possibly the only policy that will ensure the completion of the article. Besides, it is easier to write a review with the material fresh in one's mind and while inspiration is still present. I have encountered many budding authors whose only stumbling block to having an article completed was the literature review. Usually the researcher had done all the reading and taken all the notes but could not quite get around to writing the review.

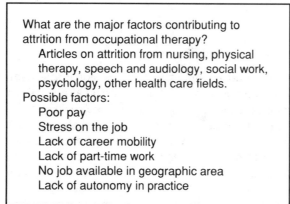

Figure 2-4 Sample card for use when searching the literature.

WORKSHEETS

Locate a convenient library.

Visit the library and familiarize yourself with the

   Card catalog
   Reference librarian
   Reference section
   Periodical room
   List of periodicals/journals stocked by that library
   Location of copying machines
   Location of nearest depository of government documents

Write your research question and main subject areas on an index card, and here:

Decide if you wish to do a hand search or a computer search:

_____ Hand   _____ Computer

If you decide on a *hand search*, decide on the indexes and abstracts that are the most appropriate for your subject (a conversation with the reference librarian might be helpful).

   Indexes and abstracts you plan to use:

If you decide on a *computer search*, decide on the data base most appropriate for your subjects (discuss with the librarian) and peruse the thesaurus for terms.

Data base: Data base:

      Terms: Terms:

Discuss the search with the librarian (costs, methods of payment, if you can be present during the search *or* mailing time if attendance is impractical) and arrange a time for the search.

When the search has been carried out, review the list of titles and abstracts generated by the computer and check off those you wish to locate.

FOR HAND *OR* COMPUTER SEARCH

Find books, articles, or dissertation abstracts and complete index cards on peripheral subjects at the library.

Make copies of important articles or abstracts. Take these home, together with books you need.

Complete index cards on all data sources.

Decide on specific subject areas. List here:

Subject A:

B:

C:

D:

E:

Group index cards into specific subject areas.

Store cards in a safe place until you are ready to write your literature review.

Write your literature review as soon as you have located and read all the items on your literature search list.

REFERENCES

American Psychological Association. (1983). *Publication manual of the American Psychological Association* (3rd ed.). Washington, DC: Author.

Bailey, D.M. (1990). Reasons for attrition from occupational therapy. *American Journal of Occupational Therapy, 44*(1), 23–29.

Beckman, C.E., & Axtell, L.A. (1987). Prosthetic use in elderly patients with dysvascular above-knee and through-knee amputations. *Physical Therapy, 67*(10), 1510–1516.

Walker, M.L., Rothstein, J.M., Finncane, S.D., & Lamb, R.L. (1987). Relationship between lumbar lordosis, pelvic tilt, and abdominal muscle performance. *Physical Therapy, 67*(4), 512–516.

ADDITIONAL READING

Berger, R.M., & Patchner, M.A. (1988). *Planning for research: A guide for the helping professions.* No. 50 in Sage Human Services Guide Series. Newbury Park, CA: Sage Publications.

Currier, D.P. (1984). Chapter 3: Literature review. In *Elements of research in physical therapy* (pp. 34–50). Baltimore: Williams & Wilkins.

Hall, M. (1987). Unlocking information technology. *American Journal of Occupational Therapy, 41*(11), 722–725.

Lehmkuhl, D. (1978). Techniques for locating, filing and retrieving scientific information. *Physical Therapy, 58*, 579–581.

Oyster, C.K., Hanten, W.P., & Llorens, L.A. (1987). Chapter 1: Foundations of health science research. In *Introduction to research: A guide for the health science professional* (pp. 1–16). Philadelphia: J.B. Lippincott.

Payton, O.D. (1988). Chapter 10: The library as a research tool. In *Research: The validation of clinical practice* (pp. 185–199). Philadelphia: F.A. Davis.

Stein, F. (1989). Chapter 5: Review of the literature. In *Anatomy of clinical research: An introduction to scientific inquiry in medicine, rehabilitation, and health related professions* (pp. 151–163). Thorofare, NJ: Slack, Inc.

Refining the Question and Developing the Background

As a way of refining the research question and developing the background, I find it helpful to start writing about the project at this juncture. Information from the literature search is still fresh in my mind, and most of the literature findings will be incorporated into the early parts of the written article. Writing the initial sections as work progresses also makes preparation for publication easier when that time comes.

THE PROBLEM

The heart of the study is the problem statement, and all other elements will flow from it. This is the reason for undertaking the study; it is the problem or question that caught your interest in the first place—the issue you wanted to solve in your clinical practice. Following the review of what has been written about the topic, it should be possible to write about the problem comprehensively. Is it a problem for many clinicians/educators/administrators? Have others identified it and tried to do something about it? Were their attempts successful or unsuccessful? What will you do differently in your attempt to solve the problem? Or are you merely trying to gather more data about it? (See Box 3–A.)

We were usually driven to action such as carrying out research by identifying something that is wrong, something that needs attention, or by old ideas or methods that are no longer adequate. The paragraph stating the problem you intend to address should be brief and to the point. Tell the reader what is wrong, what has failed, what is missing, what current ideas are presumed true that you wish to challenge, or what program needs to be scrutinized. Write two or three sentences about the problem, and read it to a colleague. If he or she misses the point, try again. Listen to yourself as you read—is this really the problem you want to do something about? (See Box 3–B.)

THE BACKGROUND

Once you are satisfied with the wording of the problem, you are ready to address the background of your study. The background answers the questions "Why is this problem of concern?" "Why is it of theoretical interest?" From your reading, you should mention why

Box 3–A

Moncur (1987) states the underlying problem for her study:

> A consensus currently exists among rheumatologists . . . and physical therapists that physical therapy should be an integral part of the treatment program of the patient with arthritis. The ability of the physical therapist to provide appropriate care to those who suffer with this group of chronic diseases has been questioned recently. In 1982, the National Arthritis Advisory Board (NAAB) reported that, because of severe budgetary restraints, the education of health care professionals in rheumatology was limited severely. The NAAB suggested that nursing and allied health professionals do not have adequate rheumatology training programs and depend on an informal process in clinical practice to learn to treat patients with arthritis. (p. 331)

Moncur talks of others' attempts to determine the adequacy of classroom and clinical exposure of physical therapists to rheumatology, then states that her approach to the problem is "to investigate what skills physical therapists and [rheumatologists] believe an entry-level physical therapist should have to treat [arthritis] patients" (p. 331).

---

other people think it is important and needs work. Opinion as well as fact can be given in the background material when it relates to the importance of the problem (e.g., a certain senator may believe that a national health scheme is of primary importance; you can quote her if it lends credence to your problem statement).

In making this section of your article ready for publication, try to make it interesting to readers. It should capture their attention and leave them agreeing that the problem is important and worthy of investigation. If readers are not captivated by this section, they may not read any further.

If you have found public statistics from government publications during your literature search, now is the time to use them (Appendix C lists sources for such data). More often than not, these types of data offer additional background information about the problem but do not have direct bearing on the specific clinical situation under investigation. For example, if the central problem concerns insufficient subsidized health care for the poor, statistics on how many poor there are in the United States and the dollar amount of the poverty line as defined by the government may be included in the background. However, the study itself might be concerned specifically with Medicaid as a partial solution to the problem. In another example, you might be studying the specific question of which health professionals should be responsible for sexuality counseling with adults with head injury, in which case it would be useful to mention the total number of such adults in the United States because they all have the potential to benefit from this service.

Box 3–B

"Occupational therapists and health administrators have long been concerned about the shortage of occupational therapists. . . . Recently, the shortage has become critical, . . . and there is increasing pressure to boost the number of therapists practicing in the field. . . .

"The attrition of occupational therapists from the work force is a major contributor to the shortage, and retention is of primary importance in keeping a viable number of therapists practicing. . . .

"The purpose of the present study was to identify why occupational therapists are leaving the field, so that we can take the necessary steps to change certain conditions that affect occupational tenure."

(Bailey, 1990; p. 23)

THE PURPOSE

A clear statement of the purpose of your study should follow the background material. Some editors prefer that the purpose be nearer the beginning of the article, in which case you can insert it immediately after the problem statement and before the background. The purpose should tell the reader what you hope to accomplish regarding the problem by carrying out your study. Be clear about this by starting the sentence, "The purpose of the research was—." Then describe your intentions. The purposes for various studies are illustrated in Boxes 3–C, 3–D, 3–E, and 3–F. At this point in your article, the reader

---

Box 3–C

In an article about student fieldwork (Neistadt & O'Reilly, 1988), the problem and background sections state that financial constraints imposed by third-party payers and staff shortages are major reasons for cancellation of student fieldwork placements and that a specific academic program has developed a new model for fieldwork (the ILS model) to address these problems. The purpose for the paper reads: "This paper will describe the background, development, implementation, and outcomes for the ILS program" (p. 782).

Box 3–D

In a study of the effects of project versus parallel groups with senior citizens (Nelson, Peterson, Smith, Boughton, & Whalen, 1988) the purpose is stated thus:

This study tries to determine (a) whether the effects of project and parallel group structure on healthy seniors differs in terms of affective responses, group climate, or directly observed measures of social interaction and (b) whether there are differences between creative and imitative activity. (pp. 24–25)

Box 3–E

In her article "Planning Playgrounds for Children with Disabilities," Stout (1988) states the purpose as follows:

Since the value of play has been well established . . . the focus of this article will be on the planning, building, and funding of adapted playgrounds and on revisions of existing playgrounds to accommodate children with various disabilities. (pp. 653–654)

Box 3–F

A review of the literature regarding perceptual-motor deficits in alcoholic patients (Van Deusen, 1989) has its purpose stated clearly in the beginning of the article:

A literature search on perceptual-motor dysfunction in alcohol abusers was conducted for the following reasons: (a) to determine what evidence links alcohol abuse with perceptual-motor dysfunction, (b) to examine the possibility that perceptual-motor function can be improved through rehabilitation programs for alcoholics, and (c) to determine whether perceptual-motor dysfunction of alcohol abusers is related to deficits in activities of daily living and is therefore relevant to occupational therapists. (p. 384)

should be able to understand what you intend to accomplish with your project and will later be able to judge whether your methodology is likely to achieve it.

THE SIGNIFICANCE

Another section of the article which can be written as a result of the literature review is the significance of the study. The significance elaborates on what your study will do to affect the problem and why your study is important. It tells what makes your purpose worth pursuing. There are many ways to address a problem — why did you choose your particular purpose? This section will justify your search; there may be other studies addressing the issue, but you have a different purpose in mind (e.g., a group of individuals may have been overlooked by other studies, and you wish to address their needs). The significance paragraph says that your study is appropriate for the research problem and that some important benefits will occur if you do it. This is the answer to the question "So what?" It gives you the chance to provide a persuasive, rational response. (See Box 3–G.)

In writing these four sections — the problem, background, purpose, and significance — you have engaged in expansive thinking. Ideas have been global and far-reaching. Now is a good moment to pull back into microscopic thinking and ask yourself, "How would I go about achieving all this? Is it feasible?" This will give you a glimpse at methodology, the reality of how you will accomplish your purpose. Different methods for conducting studies will be discussed in Chapters 4 and 5.

RESEARCH QUESTION OR HYPOTHESIS

As a result of the writing that has been done so far, the original research question or hypothesis should have become more clear. This is the time to refine and to reshape it. For example, what may have started out as the global question "What causes therapists to leave physical therapy?" now becomes the hypothesis "Physical therapists are leaving their practice because of disillusionment with the field, low pay, and lack of promotional opportunities." Rework your hypothesis until it contains all the variables you wish to study and puts them in a relationship with one another that is supported by the literature. They may have a cause-and-effect relationship; that is, one causes something else to happen. Or they may merely be correlated; that is, if one happens, the other is more (or less) likely to happen in its presence. Boxes 3–H, 3–I, and 3–J show some examples of hypotheses.

You will note that the last two studies used the *null hypotheses* format. This is a technique used when the researcher is unsure about the outcome of the study and plans to use statistical procedures to determine whether there is a statistically significant difference between the data from the two groups, and if so, in which direction the difference lies. This concept will be discussed in more detail in Chapter 8.

Box 3–G

In the study of physical therapists' competence to treat arthritic patients mentioned in Box 3–A, the author feels that her study is significant because:

> The competencies identified in this study should assist academic planners in defining clearly their curricula and in preparing the entry-level physical therapist to treat patients with rheumatic disease. Clinicians may use these competencies to measure their ability to manage treatment of their patients who suffer from arthritis.

(Moncur, 1987, p. 338)

Box 3–H

Fitts and Howe (1987) state, "The purpose of this study is to determine if there are activity patterns in cardiac patients that characterize their use of leisure." Their hypotheses are:

Hypothesis 1: Cardiac subjects spend more time in work and less time in play, rest, and/or sleep, than noncardiac subjects.
Hypothesis 2: Cardiac subjects derive less satisfaction from their leisure activities than noncardiac subjects.
Hypothesis 3: Cardiac subjects engage in fewer tension-reducing activities than noncardiac subjects.

(p. 584)

Box 3–I

A thesis investigated pinch and grip strength related to performance on a specific hand function test (Ball, 1986) and tested the null hypotheses:

1. There is no significant correlation between grip strength and hand function in the normal population.
2. There is no significant correlation between pinch strength (lateral, 2 point tip, 3 point tip, 2 point pad, 3 point pad) and hand function in the normal population.
3. Dominant hands will have a different pattern of correlation between strength and function than nondominant hands.

(p. iii)

Box 3–J

A study to examine the effort made by subjects engaged in purposeful and non-purposeful activities (Bloch, Smith, & Nelson, 1989) tested the following null hypotheses:

That there would be no significant difference between jumping with a rope and jumping without a rope on each of the following dependent variables:

- pulse rate increase from baseline to cessation of jumping,
- duration of jumping,
- ratings on each of the three factors of the Osgood Semantic Differential,
- activity preference.

(p. 27)

When you feel pleased with your hypothesis, go back to Chapter 1 and review the items that make a question realistic and researchable to be sure that yours still meets the criteria. Perhaps you will find that you now need different resources or a more refined subject pool. Rework the appropriate sections of the Chapter 1 worksheets.

STUMBLING BLOCKS

It is quite common for the researcher to confuse the problem, purpose, and significance of a study. Remember:

- The problem is the larger issue that others have tried to do something about.
- The purpose is what you hope to accomplish as a result of your small contribution to the larger problem.
- The significance is the importance of your particular study and what it will do to help solve the larger problem. It is the "So what?" of the study.

WORKSHEETS

PROBLEM STATEMENT

What is the general topic area of your project?

What is the *specific problem* you plan to address?

- Is there something wrong?
- Does something need attention?
- Is something missing?
- Do old ideas need revising?
- Do old methods need revising?
- Has something failed?
- Is there a program that needs revising?

Relate your problem statement to a colleague.

Did he/she understand it?

Is this really the problem you want to do something about?

BACKGROUND

Look at your problem statement:

Give at least three reasons why your problem is important and valid — to you, to society, to your profession.

1.

2.

3.

Specify at least two concrete examples of the problem:

1.

2.

To what public statistics, political trends, or theoretical controversy does your study relate?

PURPOSE

What do you hope to *accomplish* regarding the problem by carrying out your project?

Will you
- change something?
- understand something?
- interpret something differently?

Write the *purpose* of your study here:

Read through your purpose. Can the reader now understand what you intend to accomplish through your project? How you are going to help solve the problem?

_____ Yes
_____ No

If doubtful, restate your purpose, beginning:
    "The purpose of this study is—"

SIGNIFICANCE

Why is your study important? To whom is it important other than yourself? (Note that here you do not deal with the importance of the *problem*, but rather with the importance of the *study*.)

What can happen that will be of benefit if the study is done? What might happen if it is not done?

Write the *significance* section here:

Place yourself in the position of responding to someone who asks you, "So what?" about your project. What would be your persuasive, rational response?

REFERENCES

Bailey, D. M. (1990). Reasons for attrition from occupational therapy. *American Journal of Occupational Therapy, 44*(1), 23–29.

Ball, J. H. (1986). *Pinch and grip strength related to performance on the Jebsen Hand Function Test.* Unpublished master's thesis, Tufts University, Medford, MA.

Bloch, M., Smith, D., & Nelson, D. (1989). Heart rate, activity, duration, and affect in added-purpose versus single-purpose jumping activities. *American Journal of Occupational Therapy, 43*(1), 25–30.

Fitts, H., & Howe, M. (1987). Use of leisure time by cardiac patients. *American Journal of Occupational Therapy, 41*(9), 583–589.

Moncur, C. (1987). Perceptions of physical therapy competencies in rheumatology. *Physical Therapy, 67*(3), 331–339.

Neistadt, M., & O'Reilly, M. (1988). Independent living skills model for level 1 fieldwork. *American Journal of Occupational Therapy, 42*(12), 782–786.

Nelson, D., Peterson, C., Smith, D., Boughton, J., & Whalen, G. (1988). Effects of project versus parallel groups on social interaction and affective responses in senior citizens. *American Journal of Occupational Therapy, 42*(1), 23–29.

Stout, J. (1988). Planning playgrounds for children with disabilities. *American Journal of Occupational Therapy, 42*(10), 653–657.

Van Deusen, J. (1989). Alcohol abuse and perceptual-motor dysfunction: The occupational therapist's role. *American Journal of Occupational Therapy, 43*(6), 384–390.

ADDITIONAL READING

Berger, R. M., & Patchner, M. A. (1988). *Planning for research: A guide for the helping professions.* No. 50 in the Sage Human Service Guide Series. Newbury Park, CA: Sage Publications.

Marshall, C., & Rossman, G. B. (1989). *Designing qualitative research.* Newbury Park, CA: Sage Publications.

Deciding on Methodology

You are now ready to think about the method that will be used in your research project; that is, what design you will use to answer the question that has been posed in order to deal with the identified problem. Although there are many ways to think about and organize research methods or designs, one of the most helpful is to divide them into the following three categories:

1. True experimental designs
2. Quasi-experimental designs
3. Non-experimental designs

As listed, these designs have decreasing levels of experimental rigor but become more and more practical when it comes to human subject research, meaning that it is often difficult to achieve the standards required for true experimental designs because of the vagaries of human behavior.

By way of explanation of the above paragraph, let us look at exactly what is required for each level of design. To do this, three concepts must be explained:

1. Manipulation
2. Control
3. Randomization

MANIPULATION

Manipulation is a sinister-sounding word that has a particular meaning in research that is different from its everyday meaning. In research, it merely means doing something to the subjects in the study; for example, if the researcher offers a group of schizophrenic patients a daily program of self-care activities to see if their appearance can be improved, manipulation is being provided in the form of daily self-care activities. Generally, any therapy offered to subjects in the hope that they will show improvement can be called manipulation, using research terms.

In other words, the researcher is manipulating one or more variables in connection with the subjects, a variable being anything that can vary or change and therefore can be measured. In the above example, the variable of self-care is being manipulated or treated in the hope that it will have an effect on another variable, namely, the patients' appearance.

DEPENDENT AND INDEPENDENT VARIABLES

One other point important to understand is which variable is being manipulated. The reader has doubtless heard about dependent and independent variables. In the example above, the independent variable is manipulated (self-care) to see its effect on the dependent variable (appearance). The independent variable is sometimes called the experimental or treatment variable. The dependent variable (appearance) determines the effectiveness of the manipulation/treatment of the independent variable (self-care skills program). It is the item observed and measured at the beginning and end of the study.

Manipulation must be part of the methodology if the study is to qualify as a true experimental design. From this statement, it is plain to see that where the researcher does not actually manipulate a variable pertaining to the subjects (for example, when subjects are asked to complete a questionnaire and the researcher merely examines answers/variables after the fact and does not actually manipulate them), these are not experimental studies.

CONTROL

The second concept that needs definition in order to understand the categories of research design is that of control. Control refers to the experimenter's ability to control or eliminate interfering and irrelevant influences from the study. This will allow the researcher to say that the results are due to manipulation of the variables and not to chance interferences of other variables. In the example above, if there were no control, it is possible that some other event in the lives of the patients (such as a volunteer taking them to the store to buy new clothes) might have caused improvement in their appearance rather than the program of self-care skills.

The researcher may be able to control some variables such as (a) environmental influences (e.g., the amount of noise or the aesthetics of surroundings); (b) change of therapist providing the treatment (it might be important to the study that the same therapist be used so that patients become accustomed to him or her, or it might be equally important that different therapists be used to eliminate the influence of certain therapist styles); and (c) certain events in the patients' lives (such as obtaining a physician's cooperation in not changing patients' medications during the period of the study).

However, it is not possible to control all variables that may affect the study results, which is why it is usual to have a control group of subjects who experience the same day-to-day occurrences and influences as the experimental group but who do not receive the study treatment. By including a control group, the researcher is attempting to ensure that any helpful or detrimental event influencing the amount of change in the dependent variable (the one being measured) will happen to both groups of subjects. At the end of the study when the dependent variable is measured for both groups, if there is greater improvement in the experimental group, the researcher can say that this was probably due to the manipulation or treatment, because the control group did not receive the treatment but did experience the same day-to-day influences.

There are times when it would not be ethical to withhold treatment from a group of patients in order for them to comprise a control group. These occasions may occur when a therapist would like to know if a new form of treatment is more effective for a certain condition than the traditional treatment for that condition. In that case, the control group could receive the traditional treatment and the experimental group could receive the new treatment, and all other conditions would be held constant. This design satisfies the need for a control group as well as the ethical concern. However, there are still other occasions when it is possible to improve upon this design by adding a third group who receive no treatment at all, while experiencing the same day-to-day conditions. The results would be even more convincing if a group receiving one of the treatments showed more improvement than the non-treatment group.

It can be seen therefore, that control is about the business of eliminating influences that are not part of the study design. The concept of control actually embraces elements of the third concept to be discussed, that of randomization.

RANDOMIZATION

Randomization is designed to reduce the risk of systematic bias creeping into the study by ensuring that the subjects are representative of the group from which they are chosen and by ensuring that the experimental and control group subjects are similar. The two components are random selection of the subjects and random assignment of subjects to groups. Randomization increases (1) the internal validity of the study, which is the chance that we are actually changing and measuring what we think we are changing and measuring in a particular study, and (2) the external validity of the study, which is the chance that results found in subjects can be generalized to others who are similar (see Box 4–A). Randomly selecting subjects from a larger group of people and randomly assigning those chosen to experimental and control groups will also reduce the chance of bias in the formation of the sample groups.

Randomization has a precise meaning in research. *Random selection* means that every subject in the population concerned has an equal chance of being selected for the study sample.

The term *population* also has a specific meaning in research. It is the entire group of people or items that meet the criteria set by the researcher. Population refers to all such subjects in the world, while *subpopulation* is a defined subgroup of the population. A sample is selected from the population or from the subpopulation (see Box 4–B). In research, a population does not necessarily refer to people, but may refer to things such as records or events that are being studied, as may be seen from the example in Box 4–C.

It can be seen that if every subject in the population must have an equal opportunity of being selected, merely using as subjects patients who come through your door or client records that happen to land on your desk would mean that not all subjects had the same chance of being included in the study, because all those who did not walk through your door or whose records did not land on your desk had no chance of being selected. Instead, a complete list of people or items in the population or subpopulation must be available to the researcher and a random selection made from that list. In King's case (Box 4–B), she would have needed a complete list of all the patients in the Arizona State Hospital who met the research criteria (i.e., all those of the chronic non-paranoid–type schizophrenic). She then could have placed all the names in a hat and picked out the required number for the study, or assigned a number to each patient and used a random number chart to select patients for the study sample. Either one is an acceptable method for random selection, but the latter is probably more practical than the former.

A random number chart may be found in the back of a statistics book listing numbers that have been generated by a computer in true random fashion. The chart may be read in any direction (up or down, side to side, diagonally) starting at any point, to produce a list of random numbers. This method is commonly used when researchers are mailing questionnaires and have access to a complete mailing list of potential subjects who meet their

---

Box 4–A

If I want to change and measure the performance of mentally retarded adults on their work assembly skills and I have not randomly selected and assigned the clients, it is possible that those in the experiment (as compared with other mentally retarded adults or those in the control group) may by chance have received some work-skills training in the past, or have a greater degree of manual dexterity, or have some other trait in common of which I am not aware, any of which could make them better (or worse) at the study task.

Box 4–B

In King's study (1974) of sensory integrative therapy with schizophrenic patients, the population of interest included all the chronic, non-paranoid schizophrenic patients in the world, while the subpopulation included all the chronic, non-paranoid schizophrenic patients residing in the Arizona State Hospital. The sample for the study was selected from this subpopulation.

---

criteria—a population. It is simple enough to assign a number to each name, then to pick a series of numbers from the chart and to include the people with corresponding numbers in the study. If the list of items is already entered on a computer disk, programs are available that will make a random selection straight from the data base, saving the researcher a great deal of time.

The second component of randomization is that of randomly assigning the selected subjects to experimental and control groups. A complete subject sample should be selected first, then a similar process used to assign subjects randomly to the two groups. Random assignment to groups is primarily to ensure that the candidates in each group will be as alike (or as unalike) as possible, but also ensures that the researcher will not be tempted to assign a "good" candidate to the experimental group because it looks as if he or she will show a lot of improvement.

The point of randomization is to be sure that the sample is as representative of the population as possible and to be sure that the experimental and control groups are as similar (or as dissimilar) to each other as possible. This will enable the researcher to state more confidently that the results are due to the treatment given rather than to a difference in characteristics between the two groups, or that the sample members were not typical of the population and improved because of some uncontrolled trait that they held in common.

Random assignment will improve internal validity, that is, whether the experimental treatment made the difference rather than something else within the study design. It will even out such things as the chance of attrition between the two groups (subjects dropping out of the study); developmental maturation or practice effect having an influence on results; differences in response to testing; and regression-affecting results, such as patients getting sicker over time. On the other hand, random selection will ensure that the sample is as much like the population as possible and will therefore improve external validity, that is, that similar findings are likely if another portion of the population were studied. Thus, the results of your study can be more readily generalized to the population as a whole and are more useful to other therapists who would like to use your treatment method with similar patients. Remember, if random selection has not been used, the results of a study cannot be generalized to other people in the population.

Randomization is not perfect. It is based on the laws of probability and every once in a while the improbable will happen and a source of bias will appear in a study. For example, one group may end up being composed of patients who are sicker or older than those in the other group. Also, methods must be used correctly for random selection to be effective (see Box 4–D).

Box 4–C

In studying the effects of guided visual imagery on patients with psychosomatic, psychogenic, and chronic somatic disorders, Moore (1989) reviewed patients' charts. His subpopulation comprised all the charts of patients meeting his criteria at a specific hospital. His sample comprised 50 charts randomly selected from the subpopulation.

Box 4–D

A classic example of poor methodology occurred in the 1969 selection of men who were to be conscripted into the army. A slip of paper with name and month of birth for each man were put into an urn and drawn out, but the slips were not well mixed. The last slips put into the urn were of men whose birthdays fell in October, November, and December and disproportionately more of those men's names were drawn than others. This was a case where poor methodology resulted in serious consequences.

RESEARCH DESIGNS

Now that the concepts of manipulation, control, and randomization are understood, we can return to the requirements for the three categories of research design: true experimental designs, quasi-experimental designs, and non-experimental designs.

TRUE EXPERIMENTAL DESIGNS

In true experimental designs, all three of the concepts—manipulation, control, and randomization are required. There must be an element of control, independent variables concerning the subjects must be manipulated, and subjects must be randomly selected or randomly assigned to groups. The result is the classic experimental design that enables the researcher to say there was a good chance that the manipulation of the independent variable caused a change in the dependent variable, known as cause-and-effect research. This method allows the researcher to compare different types of treatment and to determine which type is likely to be the most effective.

In experimental research, the researcher deliberately does something to the independent variable in one group (provides a self-care training program, to use our earlier example) but not to the other (no self-care program for the control group), then looks for the results of those differences on the dependent variable (patients' appearance). The dependent variable is usually measured before and after treatment so that comparisons can be made on the same group; comparisons between groups are made by measuring both "after" tests. The before and after tests are called pre-tests and post-tests.

For ease of communication with other researchers and to permit the researcher to sketch out designs quickly, a system of shorthand known as research notation was developed by Campbell and Stanley (1969). Their system will be used throughout this book. An O represents the observations or measurements that occur at pre-testing and post-testing; an R represents random assignment; and an X represents manipulation or treatment. Each study group is written or represented on a separate line, and time periods are aligned with each other vertically. Thus, if we wished to show in research notation a design consisting of two randomly assigned groups, one with treatment and one without, and both with pre-testing and post-testing, we would show it thus:

$$R \quad O \quad X \quad O$$
$$R \quad O \qquad O$$

This is a classic experimental design and one that would be most effective in investigating the efficacy of a new treatment method. If one wanted to investigate whether or not a new treatment method were more effective than a traditional one, and if the two methods were better than no treatment at all, one could use the design mentioned earlier, where a third group is added. It would look like this in research notation:

$$R \quad O \quad X_1 \quad O$$
$$R \quad O \quad X_2 \quad O$$
$$R \quad O \qquad O$$

The two treatment groups would be differentiated by the use of subscripts 1 and 2.

As mentioned at the beginning of this chapter, in human subject research often it is not possible to provide all the requirements for experimental research (manipulation, control, and randomization). Perhaps it is impossible to randomly assign subjects to different groups (Campbell and Stanley [1969] feel that random assignment is sufficient to qualify as a true experimental research design because random selection is so difficult to achieve), or it is not ethically possible to have a control group go without treatment. In these cases, it is often necessary to move to the next category — to a quasi-experimental research design.

QUASI-EXPERIMENTAL DESIGNS

To qualify as a quasi-experimental design, it remains necessary to manipulate the independent variable in order to look for an effect on the dependent variable but either control or randomization may be lacking. The resulting designs are still very useful to clinicians looking for validation of treatment methods and techniques, but they do lack generalizability if there is no random selection, and they are open to outside influences on the results if there is no control group or no random assignment (see Box 4–E).

Sometimes researchers will use subjects as their own controls. This refers to the situation in which there is no second group who are without treatment, but rather the subjects in the experimental group themselves double as the control group. They not only receive the treatment but also experience a period of time when there is no treatment occurring, which is considered the control period. In research notation, the design looks like this:

$$O \quad X_1 \quad O \qquad O \quad X_2 \quad O \qquad O \quad X_3 \quad O$$

It can be seen that an observation pre-test occurs, and the first treatment is given, followed by a post-test. Then a similar amount of time to the treatment period elapses when no treatment is given, followed by a second post-test. This test becomes the pre-test for the second period of treatment, which now follows, and so on, until the desired number of treatment and non-treatment periods have been given. During the non-treatment period, one would not expect to see any change in the dependent variable if in fact the treatment were the influence causing change, just as one would not expect to see change in the dependent variable in a control group. If one were to draw a graph of the expected results of this research design, it would look something like the drawing in Figure 4–1.

If the results did look similar to this, it would be fairly certain that the improvement in the dependent variable was due to the treatment procedure, and that when the treatment was not occurring, subject improvement leveled off. Of course, in reality improvements are

---

Box 4–E

In Jongbloed, Stacey, and Brighton's study (1989) comparing patients' improvement following cerebral vascular accidents (CVAs), their sample comprised post-CVA patients who were admitted to a hospital in Vancouver during a specific 4-month period. The researchers randomly assigned patients to the two experimental groups, thus ensuring equivalence between the groups. For ethical reasons, they were not able to include a control or non-treatment group in their study. Instead, they provided different types of treatment to the two groups and compared results. Their research design looks like this:

$$R \quad O \quad X_1 \quad O$$
$$R \quad O \quad X_2 \quad O$$

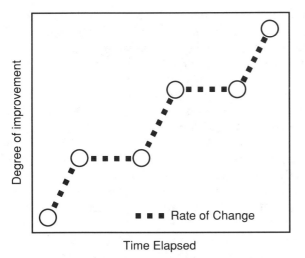

Figure 4–1 Representation of expected results when subject is used as his or her own control.

unlikely to start and stop as abruptly as the graph would indicate—there would probably be some effect of the treatment spilling over into the control period.

Having said that quasi-experimental research demands manipulation but that either control or randomization may be missing, it should be noted that there are some designs that do not have either control or randomization, yet fall into the quasi-experimental category because there is manipulation of an independent variable. The classic case is the single case experiment, that is, one subject (or group of subjects) who receives pre-test, treatment, and post-test. (Campbell and Stanley [1969] refer to this as a pre-experimental design.) There are no control subjects, and there obviously cannot be any random assignment. Research notation for this design looks like this:

$$O \quad X \quad O$$

This design is fraught with difficulties and some feel it is of little value. The pros and cons of this design will be discussed in more detail in Chapter 5, which describes research designs.

NON-EXPERIMENTAL DESIGNS

Non-experimental designs are characterized by having no manipulation of an independent variable. Control and randomization are not possible or even relevant facets of this type of research. These are usually designs in which the researcher is intending to investigate (a) a variable that cannot be manipulated or changed because it is fixed (e.g., hair color, age, and height), or (b) one that cannot be changed because it has already happened (e.g., auto accidents, drug abuse, an event in history such as a medical discovery), or (c) one in which the investigator wants to measure and compare two or more existing variables to see if there is a relationship between them (e.g., height and weight, therapist personality and patient attendance at treatment). Because the variables in all three cases are being studied after they have occurred, this type of research is often referred to as *ex post facto* (roughly translated as "after the fact") research. Non-experimental research is also called descriptive research because one is simply describing characteristics and events connected with a sample and not manipulating them in any way.

Included in the ex post facto category of designs are correlational studies where one is looking for a relationship between two or more variables, survey research using interviews or questionnaires, historical research where a historical event is studied and new interpretations evolve, ethnographic or observational studies where the researcher is immersed in the culture of the group under study, and the case study (sometimes called the single case report) where a single subject is observed and new interpretations and suggestions for treatment emerge. All of these will be discussed in the next chapter.

Perhaps while reading this chapter, you have formulated some ideas about which research design would be preferable for your project. You should first decide if your project falls into an experimental or non-experimental mode. That is, do you intend to manipulate an independent variable, to actually offer some treatment, or will you be engaged in ex post facto research where you will be investigating a variable that is fixed or already has occurred? If you are planning to provide treatment/manipulation, can you meet the other two criteria for a true experimental design — control and randomization? If not, which of the quasi-experimental designs is appropriate for your study? If you know you are doing non-experimental research, you will wish to read further about these designs before deciding which is appropriate for you. The next chapter will describe some of the actual designs used in experimental, quasi-experimental and non-experimental studies.

STUMBLING BLOCKS

One of the difficult blocks in research design is deciding which is the independent and which is the dependent variable. If the study calls for a treatment approach, the decision is relatively easy — the treatment is the independent variable. It is also obvious that the variable you hope to change is the dependent variable, the one that will be measured to look for the change.

The independent variable is one whose boundaries are defined in advance by the researcher. It is selected because it is seen as being causative or very important to the logical purpose of the research project. In cause-and-effect or experimental research, the independent variable is always the one assumed to cause something to happen, and the dependent variable is always the one being changed.

In ex post facto research, where the independent variable cannot be manipulated because it is fixed or it has already happened, it is still feasible to use the term *independent variable* and to assume that a variable is causative in nature. One usually makes this assumption based on experience and reading. However, it may not be easy to identify because it is not being manipulated by the researcher and is not easily identified as treatment.

A common mistake regarding the independent variable in non-experimental research is thinking that one can still claim a cause-and-effect relationship between independent and dependent variables. In ex post facto research, as stated earlier, the independent variable cannot be manipulated by the researcher because it is fixed or has already happened. In this case, a variable — for example, depression — is studied after the fact to see if it is likely to have affected another variable, such as productivity. Because this is not being tested in a true experimental manner, it is not possible to claim a cause-and-effect relationship, but only an associative relationship. This puts the study in the realm of correlational (non-experimental) research. Because we are not now manipulating the independent variable (depression), the results should be expressed in terms of association or relationship between variables and not in terms of cause and effect.

The true meaning of the term *random* often escapes people and they think the everyday usage of random selection, (i.e., picking people haphazardly with no apparent pattern), is the research meaning of the word. As was noted in the text earlier, the term *random* has a specific meaning in research for selection and assignment of subjects, and if the researcher does not apply correct randomization procedures, results of the study cannot be generalized to similar populations.

WORKSHEETS

Think about your project.

A. Do you intend to offer treatment to a group of patients?
   If not, go on to Section **B**.
   If so, name the treatment.

What is the independent variable that you are manipulating?

What dependent variable do you expect to change as a result?

RANDOMIZATION

Think about your subject selection criteria. What attributes have a bearing on your study (e.g., age, gender, type of disability, degree of disability, location of residence)?

Is it possible for you to obtain a list of all the individuals who meet your criteria?

       _____ In your facility?
       _____ In a group of similar facilities in your area?
       _____ Nationwide?

If so, do you know how to go about random selection and random assignment?

What method of random selection and random assignment to groups will you use?

CONTROL

Is it possible for you to have a control group of subjects?

METHODOLOGY

Based on the answers to the above questions, do you have a

True experimental design? _____

Quasi-experimental design:

Lacking randomization? _____
Lacking control? _____
Use research notation to map out your design.

B. You are doing non-experimental research.

Are you interested in studying a

_____ Variable that is fixed?
_____ Variable that has already occurred?
_____ Comparison of one or more variables that have occurred?

Name the variable(s).

REFERENCES

Campbell, D.T., & Stanley, J.C. (1969). *Experimental and quasi-experimental designs for research.* Skokie, IL: Rand McNally.

Jongbloed, L., Stacey, S., & Brighton, C. (1989). Stroke rehabilitation: Sensorimotor integrative treatment versus functional treatment. *American Journal of Occupational Therapy, 43*(6), 391–397.

King, L.J. (1974). A sensory-integrative approach to schizophrenia. *American Journal of Occupational Therapy, 28*(9), 529–536.

Moore, D.A. (1989). *Guided visual imagery as an occupational therapy modality.* Unpublished master's thesis, Tufts University, Medford, MA.

ADDITIONAL READING

Cox, R.C., & West, W.L. (1986). Chapter 4: Selecting a research design. In *Fundamentals of research for health professionals* pp. 25–45. Laurel, MD: RAMSCO Publishing Co.

Fox, J.A., & Tracy, P.E. (1989). *Randomized response: A method for sensitive surveys.* No. 58 of Quantitative Application in the Social Sciences Series. Newbury Park, CA: Sage Publications.

Kalton, G. (1989). *Introduction to survey sampling.* No. 35 of Quantitative Application in the Social Sciences Series. Newbury Park, CA: Sage Publications.

Lehmkuhl, D. (1970). Let's reduce the understanding gap: 3. Experimental design: What and why? *Physical Therapy, 50*(12), 1716–1720.

Morse, A. (Ed.) (1985). *New dimensions in research for health professionals* [Cassette recordings and workbook]. Laurel, MD: American Occupational Therapy Foundation and RAMSCO Publishing Co.

Oyster, C., Hanten, W., & Llorens, L. (1987). *Introduction to research: A guide for the health science professional.* Philadelphia: J.B. Lippincott.

Partridge, C.J., & Barnitt, R.E. (1986). Chapter 4: Research design. In *Research guidelines: A handbook for therapists* (pp. 23–35). Rockville, MD: Aspen Publishers.

Payton, O. (1988). *Research: The validation of clinical practice* (2nd ed.). Philadelphia: F.A. Davis Co.

Stein, F. (1989). Anatomy of clinical research: An introduction to scientific inquiry in medicine, rehabilitation, and health related professions. Thorofare, NJ: Slack, Inc.

Research Designs

In this chapter, some of the major research designs will be described and their advantages and disadvantages discussed. There are, of course, many more designs than are presented here, but beginning researchers should be able to find a design to fit their needs in getting started in the research process. This chapter is divided into experimental designs, quasi-experimental designs, and non-experimental designs.

EXPERIMENTAL DESIGNS

THE CLASSIC DESIGN

The classic design with experimental and control groups, random selection, pre-testing, and post-testing has already been presented in Chapter 4. In research notation, the design is represented thus:

$$R \quad O \quad X \quad O$$
$$R \quad O \quad \quad O$$

You will remember that this design provides for the three essential components of experimental research—randomization, control, and manipulation of the independent variable. Using this design, subjects are randomly selected and assigned to either an experimental or a control group. Pre-tests and post-tests are administered to both groups. The resulting data from the pre-tests will enable the researcher to see whether or not the two groups are truly alike. Post-test scores can be compared to see which group shows the greatest change in the dependent variable. Finally, the pre-test and post-test of each group can be compared to see how much change occurred for the experimental versus the control group.

If circumstances dictated, the random assignment to groups could actually be performed after the pre-test; however, the assignment should be in no way influenced by the results of the pre-test. Following random assignment, equivalency between the two groups may be assumed, yet performing a pre-test provides a further check on equivalency. This double check is particularly useful in dealing with small samples. Nevertheless, mortality (loss of participants), particularly that which is different between experimental and control groups, should be a continuing concern.

FOLLOW-UP

If you wish to know if the effect of the intervention is long-lasting, the design may be further improved by adding a follow-up observation or post-test (O_2 and O_4), thus:

$$R \quad O \quad X \quad O_1 \quad O_2$$
$$R \quad O \quad \quad O_3 \quad O_4$$

This will enable you to see if any improvement following the treatment has been maintained over time. Box 5–A illustrates the point with a follow-up observation occurring 2 months after the post-test.

OMITTED PRE-TEST

Sometimes, the results of the treatment may be influenced by the fact that a pre-test has been administered. For example, subjects may benefit from practicing a task used in the pre-test, thus diminishing the effect of the intervention. In this case, the pre-test may be omitted as long as there has been random selection and random assignment to groups. The resulting design looks like this:

$$R \quad X \quad O$$
$$R \quad \quad O$$

However, if the investigator is not sure whether or not the pre-test has an effect, or knows that it has an effect but feels that it provides crucial information, the Solomon four-group design can be employed.

SOLOMON FOUR-GROUP DESIGN

The Solomon four-group design is a powerful research design, but requires many subjects and a great deal of researcher time. It is constructed thus:

$$1. \; R \quad O \quad X \quad O_1$$
$$2. \; R \quad O \quad \quad O_2$$
$$3. \; R \quad \quad X \quad O_3$$
$$4. \; R \quad \quad \quad O_4$$

Box 5–A

A 1989 study compared

the effectiveness of excitatory and inhibitory multisensory stimulation for reducing instances of stereotypic behavior (STB) in a severely multiply disabled population. Thirty-six subjects were randomly assigned to three groups (excitatory, inhibitory stimulation, and control groups) and the two experimental groups received a treatment intervention for 30 days. . . . STB was measured before, after, and 2 months after the intervention period.

The design would have been notated thus:

$$R \quad O \quad X \quad O \quad O$$
$$R \quad O \quad X \quad O \quad O$$
$$R \quad O \quad \quad O \quad O$$

(Iwasaki & Holm, 1989, p. 170)

There is random assignment to four groups, two experimental and two control groups:

- One group receives the pre-test and the experimental treatment followed by a post-test.
- A second group is given a pre-test and a post-test but no treatment.
- The third group is not given a pre-test but receives the experimental treatment and a post-test.
- The fourth group receives only the post-test.

In comparing the post-test results, the researcher is able to not only test for differences between experimental and control groups but is also able to test for any interaction between pre-test and experimental treatment by comparing groups 1 and 3 (on O_1 and O_3) and groups 2 and 4 (on O_2 and O_4).

FACTORIAL DESIGNS

The experimental designs mentioned so far are designed to cope with one independent variable only whereas, typically, researchers are concerned with more than one variable in the same study. Factorial designs may be used to investigate two or more independent variables and their interaction with the dependent variable. These designs allow the researcher to use the same subjects to study the effects of the independent variables on the dependent variable as well as any joint effect or interaction effect. In factorial designs, each independent variable is called a factor.

For example, in Henry, Nelson, and Duncombe's study (1984) regarding choice-making in group and individual activities, the investigators wished to assess subjects' responses to having or not having choice in completing an activity. Forty subjects were divided into four groups:

1. Individual activity with choice
2. Individual activity with no choice
3. Group activity with choice
4. Group activity with no choice.

The two independent variables were: the type of activity (individual or group) and the factor of choice (choice or no choice). Therefore the study was concerned with the effects of these variables on the dependent variable—affective response. The study is charted in Figure 5–1. There are two levels for each independent variable or factor: individual and group levels for the activity factor and choice and no choice levels for the choice factor. Thus, this is called a 2×2 design.

If one of these factors had contained three levels, by adding a group who received a combination of group and individual activities for instance, it would be a 3×2 design and would be represented as shown in the chart in Figure 5–2. In a different variation, a third variable or factor, such as age, could be added to the original design with two levels for each factor, making it a $2 \times 2 \times 2$ design as depicted in Figure 5–3. Age is actually a pseudo-independent variable because it is not being manipulated by the researcher; it is an already occurring attribute of the subjects. However, in factorial designs pseudo-independent variables are often treated in the same manner as true independent variables.

	Individual activity	Group activity
Choice	Group 1	Group 2
No choice	Group 3	Group 4

Figure 5–1 Chart depicting the Henry, Nelson, and Duncombe study (1984).

	Individual	Group	Combination
Choice	1	2	3
No Choice	4	5	6

Figure 5-2 Representation of a 3×2 design.

As more variables are added, both the complexity of the design and the number of subjects required increases. Specific statistical procedures are used to analyze these designs, and usually the services of a statistician are required.

QUASI-EXPERIMENTAL DESIGNS

LACK OF RANDOMIZATION

In studying the effect of depression on self-care activities in hospitalized patients, Clark (1964) selected depressed patients from two wards and treated them as two separate groups. The design looked like this:

$$O \quad X_1 \quad O$$
$$O \quad X_2 \quad O$$

Although subjects in the two groups cannot be assumed to be equivalent because they were not randomly assigned, the researcher will have information about their pre-treatment status based on the data from the pre-tests. If they are found to be substantially different at the pre-test stage, the researcher has the choice of abandoning the groups and starting the study over, or of using statistical techniques to take into account the differences.

Convenience Samples

Major differences are likely to occur when the two groups are convenience samples, that is, groups that are already formed by some event preceding the research study. They may be groups of patients in two different wards of the same hospital, or two different nursing homes, or two day-care centers, for example. Box 5-B illustrates the use of convenience samples.

It is quite common for clinical researchers to use ready-formed groups because this is so practical. Some critics look askance at the practice, saying it is impossible to make reasonable comparisons between such groups. Others point out that using convenience samples is such a practical solution to a very real problem that we should impose whatever

Individual Activity				Group Activity			
Choice		No Choice		Choice		No Choice	
Over 50	Under 50	Over 50	Under 50	Over 50	Under 50	Over 50	Under 50
1	2	3	4	5	6	7	8

Figure 5-3 Representation of a $2 \times 2 \times 2$ design.

Name: _____ Experimental #: _____

Control #: _____

Date of birth: _____ Sex: M F

Residence: _____

Physician: _____

Diagnosis: _____

Length of time with this diagnosis: _____

Medications: Initial _____

At termination _____

Any special precautions: _____

Informed consent obtained: _____

Physician's permission to participate obtained: _____

Pre-test date: _____ Tester: _____

Post-test date: _____ Tester: _____

Treatment group attendance: X if in experimental group

C if in control group

Comments

Jan. 24 - Jan. 28 ____ ____ ____ ____ ____ _____

Jan. 31 - Feb. 4 ____ ____ ____ ____ ____ _____

Feb. 7 - Feb. 11 ____ ____ ____ ____ ____ _____

Feb. 14 - Feb. 18 ____ ____ ____ ____ ____ _____

Feb. 21 - Feb. 25 ____ ____ ____ ____ ____ _____

Feb. 28 - Mar. 4 ____ ____ ____ ____ ____ _____

Mar. 7 - Mar. 11 ____ ____ ____ ____ ____ _____

Mar. 21 - Mar. 25 ____ ____ ____ ____ ____ _____

Mar. 28 - Apr. 1 ____ ____ ____ ____ ____ _____

Apr. 4 - Apr. 8 ____ ____ ____ ____ ____ _____

Apr. 11 - Apr. 15 ____ ____ ____ ____ ____ _____

Apr. 18 - Apr. 22 ____ ____ ____ ____ ____ _____

Investigator: _____

Figure 5-4 Data collection sheet used for sensory stimulation research project.

Box 5–B

Hardison and Llorens (1988) studied the effects of a crafts group for teenage delinquent girls with suspected vestibular processing difficulties. Subjects were selected from two different group homes. Subjects from one group home became the experimental group, and subjects from the other, the control group.

---

controls we can and be alert to the variables that can impact such research. The crucial question to ask is whether the two groups truly come from the same population. The researcher may take the trouble to match subjects in the two groups so that there are commonalities in such items as socioeconomic status, gender mix, age, diagnosis, or other attributes considered important to the study. Cox and West (1986) offer a helpful description of the matching process and when it should be used. An example of matching is shown in Box 5–C.

The problem of non-representation is less likely to occur if the subjects have been randomly assigned to the research groups, even though they were not randomly selected from the target population. This obviously cannot be achieved if convenience samples are taken from different locations, but can be with a convenience sample taken entirely from one facility. Random assignment may ensure that the two groups are similar in characteristics, even though they may not be representative of the population.

Cohort Designs

When using cohort designs, a control group is again used to assess the changes made in the experimental group, but this time the groups are not observed at the same time. The groups follow each other through a setting such as classes of pupils moving through a high school or groups of trainees entering a sheltered workshop for a training period. One group is selected as the experimental group and subjected to a unique experience, while another group acts as the control group and experiences the usual events of the setting.

The subjects in these groups are obviously not randomly chosen, because the groups are naturally occurring. Nonetheless, the two groups may be considered to be somewhat similar in that they both meet the admission requirements of the setting. The design may be depicted thus:

$$O \quad X \quad O$$
$$O \qquad O$$

There are internal validity problems with this design, because of the difference in the time of the observations. History, that is, some sort of global event that has an effect on all subjects in the sample, may play a part in accounting for the differences in data from the post-tests (see Box 5–D).

Box 5–C

Bohannon (1987) used matched controls in his study to determine whether the relative muscular endurance of patients with paresis secondary to neuromuscular disorders was different from that of comparable healthy persons. The subjects were five persons with neuromuscular disorders: cauda equina lesions (2); nerve root compression (1); muscular dystrophy (1); and Guillain-Barré syndrome (1). Bohannon matched the five control subjects by sex, age, weight, height, and peak knee extension torque of lower extremity.

Box 5–D

In studying the impact of depression on self-care management in a group of hospitalized depressed patients, a therapist reported that the death of President John F. Kennedy, partway into the study, had a profound impact on the patients (Clark, 1964). She surmised that this historically tragic event compounded the results of her study.

The cohort design can be improved upon by employing recurrent institutional cycles, using three different cohorts. The design is as follows:

$$X \quad O_1$$
$$O_2 \quad X \quad O_3$$
$$O_4$$

The first group receives the experimental treatment followed by a post-test; the second group receives the traditional pre-test, treatment and post-test; and the third group receives only a pre-test. The ideal pattern of results from this design would be similarity of responses on pre-tests O_2 and O_4 and on post-tests O_1 and O_3. The effect of the treatment would be evident by comparing scores on pre-test O_2 and post-test O_3.

LACK OF CONTROL

Time-series designs have no control group, and the subjects in the experimental group act as their own control.

Single-Group Time-Series Design

In the single-group time-series design, subjects are given a pre-test followed by experimental treatment and a post-test. A period of time is allowed to elapse, equivalent to the experimental treatment time, followed by another post-test. Periods of treatment and non-treatment are alternated with tests. During the treatment periods, the subjects in the group comprise an experimental group, and during the non-treatment periods, they are acting as a control group. Thus we have the commonly used expression "acting as their own control," which was mentioned in Chapter 4. The design is notated as follows:

$$O \quad X \quad O \qquad O \quad X \quad O \qquad O \quad X \quad O$$

The group may be randomly selected to increase the likelihood of their being representative of the population under study. Of course, the issue of random assignment to groups is a moot point, since there is only one group. This design provides a high degree of internal validity, meaning that one can be fairly sure that any changes that occur in the dependent variable at post-test are due to the experimental treatment.

Follow-up

In a variation of the time-series design, a researcher may wish to assess the permanence of change in the dependent variable and may do so by administering several post-tests after the intervention, thus:

$$O \quad X \quad O_1 \quad O_2 \quad O_3 \quad O_4$$

However, this design does have a flaw in that it is difficult to know if improvement at the first post-test (O_1) was due to the intervention or to something else including: 1) some other event that occurred concurrently; 2) something special that occurred with the procedure, instrument, or therapist; or 3) an inherent characteristic in the subject such as a seasonal improvement. There is no subsequent treatment period to use as a test for these possibilities.

Multiple Pre-tests

A third possible design of the time-series type will control for some of these flaws:

$$O \quad O \quad O \quad O \quad X \quad O \quad O \quad O \quad O$$

The multiple pre-tests will give a more accurate picture of how subjects score on the dependent variable prior to the experimental treatment, will control for seasonal or cyclical changes in abilities, and will eliminate the effect of history. An even preferable design would be:

$$O \quad O \quad O \quad O \quad X \quad O_1 \quad X \quad O_2 \quad X \quad O_3 \quad O_4 \quad O_5 \quad O_6$$

Here history is controlled for, the effects of experimental treatment can be viewed on more than one occasion (at O_1, O_2, and O_3), and the permanence of the effect can be measured (O_3 through O_6). The disadvantages of this design are that it is often impractical to wait long enough to administer several pre-tests before treating the patient and that the entire study becomes lengthy (see Box 5–E).

In spite of the fact that these are quasi-experimental designs, they are effective and can be quite practical for the clinical researcher. It is sometimes easier to gain permission to include patients in quasi-experimental studies than experimental studies. For example, it is difficult to deny treatment to patients in control groups. And finally, the fact that these designs are carried out in clinical settings with all the concomitant interferences and lack of control inherent in such settings, makes them more likely to be generalizable to other clinical settings. It is, after all, in day-to-day clinical practice that we wish to put the results of research into effect.

NON-EXPERIMENTAL DESIGNS

The nature of problems in the health sciences usually prevents the investigator from inducing causal effects. Various forms of disability and illness are frequently the target of study, and the rehabilitation professional has access to people only *after* they have acquired the disability or illness—we are not in the business of inducing disability. There-

---

Box 5–E

Ottenbacher (1982) uses a variation of the time-series analysis in his study of the effects of a sensory stimulation program and resultant duration of post-rotary nystagmus on three learning disabled children. He used a period of 5 weeks to gather baseline data on their post-rotary nystagmus, then alternately treated and tested the children over 20 weeks. They received treatment three times per week and were tested twice per week, so the resulting design looked approximately like this:

$$O\,O\,O\,O\,O \quad X\,O\,X\,O\,X \quad X\,O\,X\,O\,X \quad \ldots\ldots \quad X\,O\,X\,O\,X$$

fore, ex post facto designs must be employed. Non-experimental designs are many and varied. A representative sampling will be reviewed here.

CORRELATIONAL RESEARCH

The majority of non-experimental studies in rehabilitative health care fall in the correlational category. Correlational research is similar to experimental research in that a hypothesis is being tested; however, it is different in that there is no manipulation of independent variables, and a cause-effect relationship is not being simulated. Instead, in correlational research, the investigator is looking for a relationship between variables. Rather than hypothesizing, for instance, that being blind will cause an individual to have heightened tactile sensitivity, one might conjecture that there simply is a relationship between the variables blindness and heightened tactile sensitivity. Parenthetically, blindness has already occurred by the time the researcher is studying it, making this, de facto, "after the fact" or non-experimental research.

The researcher tests a hypothesis, comparing two or more variables by measuring differences and looking for a relationship. The procedure for the correlational research design is similar to that for experimental designs, that is: reviewing the literature, formulating research questions or hypotheses, deciding whether the hypotheses should be directional or null hypotheses, defining and operationalizing terms, selecting a sample from a population, and selecting data collection and interpretation methods.

In correlational research, however, there are specific statistical tests used for data analysis that look for an association between the two variables. This association is known as a correlation coefficient and yields a value between -1 and $+1$, where 0 indicates no relationship and the two extremes indicate a perfect negative (or inverse) relationship (-1) or a perfect positive (or direct) relationship ($+1$) (see Box 5–F).

Because this is non-experimental research and, therefore, is not subjected to the stringent rules of experimental research, similar results need to be found in many studies before therapists can claim relationships between variables concerning their patients.

SURVEY RESEARCH

Surveys are used frequently to gather information about a large population in order to answer a set of hypotheses. They are cross-sectional in the sense that they generally describe the group at one point in time, and they are used to measure the "what is" about a group rather than providing information on "why" (Cox & West, 1986). Information collected in survey research covers a vast array of topics and may include items from attitudes, values, opinions, motives, and levels of information to concrete information on such things as the respondents' work situation, environment, living situation, behaviors, and so on.

To qualify as research, the survey must be carefully crafted to answer a well-defined set of questions that have been grounded in a literature review and have significance and relevance. The manner of analysis and interpretation of the data also make this a research design rather than solely a status survey to elicit some facts about a particular group. The

---

Box 5–F

A correlational study was conducted by Short-DeGraff, Slansky, and Diamond (1989) to see if there was a relationship between preschoolers' self-drawings and results on the Goodenough-Harris Draw-a-Person Test (DAPT) and the General Information subtest of the Wechsler Preschool and Primary Scale of Intelligence (WPPSI). High correlations were obtained between the man, woman, and man/woman converted scores of the DAPT and the self-drawings ($r = .93$ and $r = .91$). Low correlations were found between all of the figure drawing and WPPSI scores (average $r = .3$).

Box 5–G

In Bailey's study (1990) on reasons for attrition from occupational therapy, she defined her population as female certified occupational therapists who were no longer working as occupational therapists. She selected her sample randomly from a) those female occupational therapists who had completed the 1986 AOTA Member Data Survey saying that they were not currently working, b) from those who had let their AOTA membership lapse, and c) from therapists whose names had been provided by colleagues because they were working in non-occupational therapy jobs.

method of analysis needs to be chosen and applied judiciously; interpretations and application to the population must be made with care.

Information may be collected either directly through a face-to-face interview or telephone interview, or indirectly through the mail or private completion of a questionnaire. These forms of data gathering are discussed in Chapter 7.

It is crucial that the relevant population is defined clearly and that their characteristics and limits are described. Sample selection methods must assure representation because the method generally used in conducting survey research is the drawing of conclusions about a large group from a smaller sample of persons (see Box 5–G). If you are not confident that the sample is representative of the population, the resulting discussion will be invalid for the larger group to whom you are generalizing.

Methods of selection, or sampling, are of crucial importance in survey research. They are described in Chapter 4 of this book. Also, Kalton's *Introduction to Survey Sampling* (1983) offers an excellent overview of methods to use when sampling for a survey.

CASE STUDY RESEARCH

In a case study, an individual, unit, or event is studied in great depth over time—anywhere from a few weeks to several years. Thus, it is a longitudinal study rather than the cross-sectional study of the survey type. Although the case being studied is often an individual person or event, it may also be a unit such as a family, a hospital ward, or a nursing home. Data may be gathered by one or more researchers through interviews, inspection of documentation, and observations. Data are gathered at various points throughout the life of the case and usually occur in a natural or real-life setting.

There has traditionally been criticism of case study research, critics citing lack of rigor in methods used, biased views influencing the direction of the findings, and the fact that it is impossible to generalize from a single case. In fact, some very fine research has been generated from case studies (Freud's and Piaget's studies being notable among others) and the criticisms can be contested. Researchers are capable of exerting controls over their tendencies toward bias and can use rigorous investigation methods.

Case studies are generalizable to theoretical propositions, rather than to populations or universes in the way that experiments are. In this sense, the case study does not represent a "sample" and the investigator's goal is to expand and generalize theories rather than to enumerate frequencies. Case studies have been used very effectively in the rehabilitation literature and have provided accounts of treatment techniques and procedures that have been helpful to therapists in their practice. The regular Case Reports section of the *American Journal of Occupational Therapy* has been especially helpful in this regard.

Case studies often fall in the category of exploratory studies, those which have as their goal the generation of hypotheses for further study under experimental conditions. In trying to decide whether to use a case study rather than one of the other types of exploratory studies such as surveys, historical studies, ethnographic studies, or archival analysis, it is useful to bear in mind that "how" and "why" questions are best answered by case studies. For example, Stein and Nikolic (1989) asked "How could a stress management training program be used to assist a young man with schizophrenia control his anxiety?"

Therapists often ask how and why a particular adaptive aid or treatment procedure worked with a particular patient. For instance, Rogers, Marcus, and Snow (1987) asked "Why did their sensory training program work with a severely regressed elderly patient?" This case illustrates the essential points of the case study approach so well that it is included in a lengthy Box—Box 5–H.

In carrying out a case study, you are looking for operational links that need to be traced over time, that is, how events are tied together to form an eventual network for successful treatment. As implied previously, case studies may be generalized to theoretical propositions and not to populations. The investigator's goal is to expand and generalize theory rather than to list occurrences of an event in order to indicate that a sample is representative of a population. In the example in Box 5–H, the authors wanted to generate theory about the role of sensory training in putting severely regressed elderly patients in touch with their environment rather than enumerating the times or the degree to which "Maude" was able to respond to the activities.

Investigators sometimes wonder when to use a single case study rather than a multi-case study. Use single case studies if:

1. you can identify *the* critical case that illustrates all the propositions of the study
2. one case is the extreme or unique case and there are no others easily available
3. you have a revelatory case that was previously unavailable to researchers
4. it is being used as a pilot study case for the multicase study approach. (Yin, 1989)

Use a multicase study approach if:

1. you want a more robust outcome
2. you have the opportunity of more than one similar case. You should adopt replication logic (i.e., all cases should be as similar as possible and you should expect to obtain similar outcomes). If you get very different findings, you need to rethink the original theory for the study. (Yin, 1989)

Box 5–H

In a case report in the *American Journal of Occupational Therapy* (1987) Rogers, Marcus, and Snow recount the story of Maude, a 90-year-old woman diagnosed with senile dementia and many other ailments such as gout, hypertension, head injury, depression, and possible cancer. Maude was non-ambulatory, incontinent, dependent for all her self-care needs, and spent most of her day non-responsive, sitting with her eyes closed. She had been a resident of a facility for many years and represented the severely regressed, sensorily deprived elderly patients with whom the authors were concerned.

Maude received an intensive sensory training program, 4 days a week for 5 weeks. The daily greeting procedure and ten core activities of the program are described in detail, together with supplementary stimulation activities and concluding procedures. Maude made dramatic gains as a result of the program. She showed a consistent increase in independent functioning during the sessions, in all ten core activities. Her initial belligerence and hostility toward the leader subsided and was replaced by open affection. She became meaningfully talkative, initiated conversations with the leader, and made comments about other participants. At the end of the program, she had become oriented to person and place, was able to look at the examiner when addressed, could respond to questions with short appropriate phrases, and showed appropriate facial expressions. Similar improvements were noted by other staff members at the facility and her gains lasted for the year during which follow-up was done.

In the discussion, the authors provide several hypotheses, conjecturing that Maude's increase in interaction may have promoted additional stimulation from staff because they found her easier to communicate with and more rewarding to be with; they hypothesize about sensory training being based on the concept that deficiencies in physical and mental stimulation contribute to cognitive impairment; and about the common characteristics of sensory deprivation seen in normal individuals. Finally, the investigators give information about the specific activities that appeared most helpful in the treatment sessions.

If you chose the multicase study approach, how many cases should you use? If there are not too many variables under study, use two or three cases; if there are many variables, increase to five or six cases. It is very appropriate to use a pilot study case for a multicase study and use it to revise such things as choice of subject, method of data collection, and type of data collected. It is not appropriate to change the original purpose or intent of the study.

The criterion for a successful case study is that theoretical propositions or hypotheses have resulted that can be tested in an experimental manner. Ultimately, the hope is that the hypotheses will be supported and give indications that will allow therapists to prescribe specific treatments for appropriate clients/patients.

Data Gathering for Case Studies

Data for the case study may be gathered in various ways. If interviews or questionnaires are used, the questions need to be carefully thought out in advance and pilot tested. If others are to administer the interview questions, they need to be trained so that questions are asked in a similar manner by all interviewers and so that correct responses to situations that may arise are rehearsed.

Documentary evidence is likely to be relevant to your case study and can take many forms. For instance, it may consist of patients' charts, minutes of meetings, reports of case presentations, patients' assessments or progress reports, or even news clippings, letters, and administrative memoranda.

Another way of gathering information is through direct observation. In making a visit to the case study "site," you may observe firsthand such things as the patient's behavior, the condition of an orthosis, or the aesthetics of the environment. By photographing, audiotape recording, and videotape recording actual places, events, and items, you will have on hand some extremely valuable records. Otherwise, it is helpful for the sake of accuracy to have more than one observer.

In analyzing the evidence you have gathered for the case study, it is important to have a strategy. Analyzing data consists of examining, categorizing, tabulating, or otherwise recombining the evidence so as to address the initial propositions of the study. Three types of techniques for analyzing case study data are pattern matching, explanation building and time-series analysis. These three methods will be described in Chapter 7.

Case studies are a useful and fascinating way for therapists to learn the investigation process. Most of us have at least one client whose progress and style of learning could benefit others, while the case study process itself requires discipline and is thought provoking.

ETHNOGRAPHY

The ethnographic style of research is one that originated in the field of anthropology and has occasionally been borrowed by health scientists to describe such settings as hospitals, special schools, sheltered workshops, and group homes. Whether or not ethnography as a research method has a place in the health sciences has been addressed by two therapists. Schmid (1981) states that "among health professionals there has been a growing interest in a research paradigm that is responsive to questions of a holistic nature, questions that generate complex knowledge about how an individual, for example a client, perceives himself and the environment in which he selects his mode of life and adapts to it" (p. 105). She goes on to say that the paradigm found in anthropology, sociology, and social psychology that emphasizes an understanding of the meaning of human behavior in social and cultural settings can satisfy such an interest. She points out that such research has been called qualitative, ethnographic, or phenomenological—it is called ethnographic in this text.

Litterst (1985) has called for a second look at the use of anthropological fieldwork methods and the concept of culture in occupational therapy research and feels that "Occupational therapists as participants in the social process of therapy are in an excellent position to formulate research projects that use fieldwork methods and expand on the dynamic elements in both occupational therapy theory and anthropological concepts of culture." (p. 604)

An ethnography attempts to be holistic, to cover as much territory as possible about a culture, a subculture, or a program. The success or failure of an ethnography depends on the degree to which it rings true to the natives—those who reside in the setting being described. The ethnographer's job is to collect information from the insider's perspective, to make sense of the data, and to offer an explanation of the workings of the whole system.

Many data-gathering techniques, including observation and participant observation, are employed that generate extensive field notes. These include structured and unstructured interviews, audiotape and videotape recordings, films and photographs, projective techniques, and techniques specific to certain types of situations such as asking participants to rank order people in their community or to rate concepts on certain rating scales. You also might use archival records such as service records, organizational charts, budgets, maps, lists of names, survey data such as census records, and personal data such as diaries, calendars, and telephone listings.

Perhaps the most difficult part of ethnographic research is making sense of the data. First, there can be enormous amounts of data to organize, and second, the data can be extremely disparate and complex. The researcher must probe topics by comparing and contrasting and trying to fit pieces of data into the larger puzzle. Specific methods for sorting, organizing, and analyzing ethnographic data will be discussed in Chapter 7.

Maps, flowcharts, organizational charts, and matrices can provide visual representations of an ethnographer's understanding of a community. They all help to crystallize and display information and are useful in an analysis.

Ethnographers crystallize their thoughts at various stages throughout a study. The crystallization may bring a mundane conclusion, a novel insight, or an earth-shattering awakening. Crystallization is typically the result of a convergence of similarities that strike the researcher as important to the study. Every study has classic moments when everything falls into place, a special configuration gels. This is usually when all forms of analysis have been completed and layers of triangulated effort, key events, and patterns of behavior form a coherent picture, and this is when the work of the study has been achieved (see Boxes 5–I and 5–J).

METHODOLOGICAL RESEARCH

For many years, therapists have been interested in developing and fabricating their own adaptive aids, equipment, tests, and other instruments for use in the evaluation and

---

Box 5–I

Perhaps the most thorough ethnographic study of occupational therapy to date has occurred as a result of the Clinical Reasoning Study co-sponsored by the American Occupational Therapy Foundation and the AOTA (1986–1990). The methods used by the researchers were the traditional methods of ethnography, the lead researcher being an anthropologist. Researchers used videotaped recordings of experienced and novice occupational therapists treating patients in the clinical environment, together with participant observation and in-depth interviewing. They analyzed the tapes using chunking (allowing the researchers to find patterns in the interactions) and comparative analysis (described in Chapter 7 of this book), which resulted in hypothesis generation and grounded theory about the clinical reasoning used by therapists. Some results of the study are reported by Fleming (1989), Gillette and Mattingly (1987), and Mattingly (1988, 1989a, 1989b).

> **Box 5–J**
>
> The abstract of Krefting's (1989) study on the reintegration into the community of 21 head-injured persons, mentions the ethnographic data collection and data analysis methods used.
>
> This paper reports the findings of an ethnographic study of 21 moderately head-injured persons living in the community and of their social networks. Three fieldwork strategies were used to collect the data: semistructured interviews, participant observation, and documentary review. The data were subjected to thematic and content analysis. A portion of the findings is described in terms of recasting strategies, which are linked to a theoretical concept of loss of self-identity and personhood. . . .
>
> (p. 67)

treatment of their patients. They wish to test and improve the validity and reliability of such materials, and methodological research methods may be used to achieve these goals. Methodological research develops, validates, evaluates, and produces standardized measures. If the instruments used in clinical research are reliable and valid, the researcher can have more confidence in the results of the research and results can be compared across studies.

The precise set of procedures used in standardizing measures is described by Benson and Clark (1982) in their article, *A Guide for Instrument Development and Validation*. An outline of the stages includes:

1. Deciding on the purpose of the measure and the population of concern (such conditions as age, gender, diagnosis, symptomatology, place of residence, vocational goals, and psychological attributes)
2. Elucidating the content of the measure by using personal experience, review of relevant literature, and opinions of experts in the field
3. Organizing and compiling the content into a logical and meaningful sequence
4. Testing the resulting measure on a large sample of the chosen population
5. Subjecting the results to statistical tests for reliability and validity
6. Improving the design and content of the measure based on the findings
7. Retesting the measure
8. Repeating the last four steps several times until one is satisfied with the results
9. Writing an accompanying manual outlining the research process used, the population for whom the measure is intended, the results of the tests for reliability and validity, and exact procedures for using the measure.

As you can readily see from this list, "methodological research develops, validates, and evaluates standardized measures. Such research establishes the validity and reliability of research instruments, which improves the quality of research" (Oyster, Hanten, & Llorens, 1987, p. 97) by allowing us to feel more confident that we are measuring what we mean to be measuring in our studies. We often use self-made instruments in research studies without showing sufficient concern or caution in interpreting data produced by such non-standardized measures. As Oyster and colleagues (1987) point out, ". . . it is important to recognize that [methodological research] may be one of the most significant contributors to the evolution of health science research as an exact science" (p. 98).

HISTORICAL RESEARCH

Historical research is "undertaken in order to test hypotheses or to answer questions concerning causes, effects, or trends relating to past events that may shed light on present behaviors or practices" (Polit & Hungler, 1987, p. 202). Current behaviors or attitudes can often be better understood if the past is reviewed and re-examined in the light of ongoing events.

The guiding principles for historical research are the same as those for any other form of research, namely, proposing a research problem, stating guiding questions, collecting data, interpreting the results, and arriving at conclusions and implications. The main difference between historical and other types of research is that in historical research the guiding questions serve as the purpose for collecting data and the literature review provides the data, whereas in experimental research the literature review generates the questions and hypotheses. Schwartz and Colman (1988) offer an interesting article discussing the process and methods of historical research that may be used in the health sciences.

Data collection for historical research relies on primary and secondary sources, primary sources consisting of firsthand information such as autobiographies and eyewitness accounts, and secondary sources being accounts about the event not based on direct experience. The authenticity of material must be carefully evaluated. Evaluation may be achieved using external criticism—determining the authenticity or validity of the source—and internal criticism—evaluating the truth of what is said in the authentic document.

A major problem in historical research is the availability of materials for data, that is to say, the sampling. It is wise to employ as many primary sources as possible, although this is not easy because by their nature materials being studied for historical research have been destroyed and lost over time. The fact that only some of the material or evidence concerning an event is available to the researcher of history is considered a source of bias in the research design.

The data from an historical event must be critically analyzed by the researcher before any conclusions or generalizations can be made. Every document and piece of evidence must be examined with a skeptical eye, seeking substantiating proof for authorship and accuracy of content. If it is to be taken seriously, historical research must be conducted rigorously.

EVALUATION RESEARCH

Evaluation research is designed to determine: first, how a new program should be developed and designed and second, how well an existing program is doing and what should be done, if anything, to improve it. Thus, the results of evaluation research will provide answers to the questions, "What should we do?" and "How well are we doing?"

The first part is formative research, in that it represents a collection of data or opinion that can be used to form a policy upon which to design a program. Data and opinions are collected from both the users and the providers of the program.

The second part is summative research, where an existing program and its policies are evaluated. It is usual to write the program goals and objectives in behavioral terms, then to collect evidence in the form of data, to determine if the goals and objectives are being met. It is quite difficult to write goals and objectives in behavioral and measurable terms, but this is essential if the data are to be used to evaluate the effectiveness of the program.

Data are gathered from many sources including, past and present consumers of the program, representatives of all levels of providers in the program, written policies and procedures, client records, and the physical plant and its equipment. There are often large quantities of data that need to be organized and applied to each of the program's stated goals and objectives. The evaluator then must make judgments as to whether or not the goals and objectives are being met (see Box 5–K).

A program evaluator is often employed from outside the program, the advantages being that the evaluator is more likely to be objective about the program's good and bad points and is free from the burden of implementing recommended changes. If evaluators knew that they would have to make the required changes at the end of an evaluation, they might be biased in the type of changes being recommended.

Box 5–K

A study was conducted to assess the effectiveness of an occupational therapy program in the treatment of alcohol and drug dependency (Stensrud & Lushbough, 1988). The program was viewed as a demonstration project. If it was deemed successful, occupational therapy would be incorporated into the Alcohol and Drug Dependency Treatment Center.

Some examples have been provided of designs that may be employed in the three categories of research—experimental, quasi-experimental, and non-experimental. Naturally, there are many more types of research than have been mentioned here. Some further designs can be found in the *Additional Reading* list at the end of this chapter. In particular, there are many variations on the basic themes presented in the experimental and quasi-experimental categories. Careful reading of such texts as Campbell and Stanley's *Experimental and Quasi-experimental Designs for Research* (1969) and Kerlinger's *Foundations of Behavioral Research* (1979) will guide investigators toward the best design for their specific sets of circumstances.

WORKSHEETS

If you are doing experimental or quasi-experimental research and you did not find a suitable research design in the last chapter, look through the designs presented in Chapter 5 and choose the most appropriate for your project.

EXPERIMENTAL RESEARCH

a. The classic:
```
R  O  X  O
R  O     O
```

b. With follow-up:
```
R  O  X  O  O
R  O     O  O
```

c. Omitted pre-test:
```
R     X  O
R        O
```

d. Solomon four-group:
```
R  O  X  O
R  O     O
R     X  O
R        O
```

e. Factorial designs:

_____ How many factors?

_____ How many levels for each factor?

Plot out the independent variables in a table so that you can see what your design will look like:

QUASI-EXPERIMENTAL RESEARCH

a. Lack of random   O X O   or   O X O
    assignment: O X O   O   O

b. Cohort designs: O X O
                     O   O

c. Recurrent institutional
    cycles:

               X   O
                   O X O
                         O

d. Lack of control: O X O   O X O   O X O

e. With follow-up: O X O O O O

f. Multiple pre-tests: O O O O X O O O O

            or: O O O O X O X O X O O O

NON-EXPERIMENTAL RESEARCH

If you decided that your project is best suited for a non-experimental design, review the methods offered and choose the most appropriate:

a. Correlational
b. Survey
c. Case Study
d. Ethnographic
e. Methodological
f. Historical
g. Evaluation

WRITING THE RESEARCH PROTOCOL

Now it is time to operationalize the design you have chosen by writing a research protocol. In other words, you need to insert your specific variables, subjects, and procedures into the research design, creating a personalized road map for carrying out the project.

Let us say you have chosen the classic experimental design to test your hypothesis, you must now insert the method of random selection and assignment you plan to use, the criteria you will use to select subjects, your definition of dependent and independent variables, exact procedures you will use for the experimental treatment, and the exact procedures you will use to observe/pre-test and post-test the dependent variable(s).

The following is a sample of a research protocol used for a study of verbalization in patients with chronic schizophrenia (Bailey, 1978):

Subject Selection Criteria. Adult (18 years or older), male and female, chronic (diagnosed as schizophrenic for 5 years or more), non-paranoid (chart diagnosis) schizophrenic (chart diagnosis) patients (residents of an institution).

Method of Selection. Subjects will be randomly selected from two subpopulations of nursing home residents who meet the selection criteria. One group will form the experimental group and the other will form the control group.

Hypotheses. That sensory stimulation, with emphasis on vestibular input, will increase the quantity, quality, and speed of response of verbalization in chronic, non-paranoid schizophrenic adults.

Dependent Variable. The quantity, quality, and speed of response of verbalization.

Independent Variable. Sensory stimulation program with emphasis on vestibular input.

Procedures for Treatment. Administer a planned, graded program of sensory stimulation with emphasis on vestibular stimulation, to all subjects in the experimental group for:

> half-an-hour per day
> 5 days per week
> for 12 weeks.

The program will be provided in the same room of the nursing homes (the day room) each day, using a variety of sensory equipment. The group will be led by the same therapist each day, assisted by occupational therapy students.*
The control group will attend a sedentary crafts program (with as little vestibular input as possible), for the same amount of time, in the same room, led by the same staff as the experimental group.*

PROCEDURES FOR OBSERVATION

Pre-test: Individual subjects in experimental and control groups will be asked 17 questions, and their responses will be audiotape-recorded. The tester will be a person unknown to all subjects and not involved in the activity groups.

The following items will be measured using the tape recordings:

1. Number of words used in response to all questions
2. Quality of speech (as specified on attached sheet)†
3. Length of time from end of question to beginning of response (measured in seconds by stop watch).

Post-test: Individual subjects in experimental and control groups will be asked the same 17 questions as in the pre-test, and their responses will be audiotape-recorded. The tester will be the same person as was used for the pre-test. The same measurements for quantity, quality, and speed of response will be used.

Figure 5-4 (on p. 56) illustrates the data collection sheet used in this project.

---

*The actual programs for the sensory stimulation group and the craft group were written in detail for each session.
†A specific checklist for "grading" quality of speech was provided to the tester.

REFERENCES

Bailey, D. M. (1978). The effects of vestibular stimulation on verbalization in chronic schizophrenics. *American Journal of Occupational Therapy, 32,* 445–450.

Bailey, D. M. (1990). Reasons for attrition from occupational therapy. *American Journal of Occupational Therapy, 44*(1), 23–29.

Benson, J., & Clark, F. (1982). A guide for instrument development and validation. *American Journal of Occupational Therapy, 36*(12), 789–800.

Bohannon, R. W. (1987). Relative dynamic muscular endurance of patients with neuromuscular disorders and of healthy matched control subjects. *Physical Therapy, 67*(1), 18–20.

Campbell, D. T., & Stanley, J. C. (1969). *Experimental and quasi-experimental designs for research.* Chicago, IL: Rand McNally and Company.

Clark, R. (1964). *The effect of depression on self-care management.* (Unpublished paper).

Cox, R., & West, W. (1986). *Fundamentals of research for health professionals.* Laurel, MD: RAMSCO Publishing Co.

Fleming, M. (1989). The therapist with the three track mind. In *The AOTA Practice Symposium Guide.* Rockville, MD: American Occupational Therapy Association.

Gillette, N., & Mattingly, C. (1987). Clinical reasoning in occupational therapy. *American Journal of Occupational Therapy, 41*(6), 399–400.

Hardison, J., & Llorens, L. A. (1988). Structured craft group activities for adolescent delinquent girls. *Occupational Therapy in Mental Health, 8*(3), 101–117.

Henry, A., Nelson, D., & Duncombe, L. (1984). Choice making in group and individual activity. *American Journal of Occupational Therapy, 38*(4), 245–251.

Iwasaki, K., & Holm, M. B. (1989). Sensory treatment for the reduction of stereotypic behaviors in persons with severe multiple disabilities. *Occupational Therapy Journal of Research, 9*(3), 170–183.

Kalton, G. (1983). *Introduction to survey sampling.* No. 35 of Quantitative Applications in Social Sciences Series. Newbury Park, CA: Sage Publications.

Kerlinger, F. (1979). *Foundations of behavioral research.* New York: Holt, Rinehart & Winston, Inc.

Krefting, L. (1989). Reintegration into the community after head injury: The results of an ethnographic study. *Occupational Therapy Journal of Research, 9*(2), 67–83.

Litterst, T. A. (1985). The Foundation. A reappraisal of anthropological fieldwork methods and the concept of culture in occupational therapy research. *American Journal of Occupational Therapy, 39*(9), 602–604.

Mattingly, C. (1988). Perspectives on clinical reasoning for occupational therapy. In *Mental health focus: Skills for assessment and treatment.* Rockville, MD: American Occupational Therapy Association.

Mattingly, C. (1989a). *Thinking with stress: Story and experience in a clinical practice.* Doctoral dissertation, Massachusetts Institute of Technology, Cambridge, MA.

Mattingly, C. (1989b). Clinical reasoning in occupational therapy. In *The AOTA Practice Symposium Guide.* Rockville, MD: American Occupational Therapy Association.

Ottenbacher, K. (1982). Patterns of postrotary nystagmus in three learning disabled children. *American Journal of Occupational Therapy, 36*(10), 657–663.

Oyster, C. K., Hanten, W. P., & Llorens, L. A. (1987). *Introduction to research: A guide for the health science professional.* Philadelphia, PA: J.B. Lippincott.

Polit, D., & Hungler, B. (Eds.) (1987). *Nursing research: Principles and methods.* Philadelphia: J.B. Lippincott.

Rogers, J. C., Marcus, C. L., & Snow, T. L. (1987). Maude: A case of sensory deprivation. *American Journal of Occupational Therapy, 41*(10), 673–676.

Schmid, H. (1981). The Foundation. Qualitative research and occupational therapy. *American Journal of Occupational Therapy, 35*(2), 105–106.

Schwartz, K. B., & Colman, W. (1988). Historical research methods in occupational therapy. *American Journal of Occupational Therapy, 42*(4), 239–244.

Short-DeGraff, M. A., Slansky, L., & Diamond, K. E. (1989). Validity of preschoolers' self-drawings as an index of human figure drawing performance. *Occupational Therapy Journal of Research, 9*(5), 305–315.

Stein, F., & Nikolic, S. (1989). Teaching stress management techniques to a schizophrenic patient. *American Journal of Occupational Therapy, 43*(3), 162–169.

Stensrud, M. K., & Lushbough, R. S. (1988). The implementation of an occupational therapy program in an alcohol and drug dependency treatment center. *Occupational Therapy in Mental Health, 8*(2), 1–15.

Yin, R. K. (1989). *Case study research: Design and methods.* No. 5 of Applied Social Research Methods Series. Newbury Park, CA: Sage Publications.

ADDITIONAL READING

Block, J. (1971). *Understanding historical research: A search for truth.* Glen Rock, NJ: Research Publications.

Brooks, P. C. (1969). *Research in archives: The use of unpublished primary sources.* Chicago, IL: University of Chicago Press.

Converse, J., & Presser, S. (1986). *Survey questions: Handcrafting the standardized questionnaire.* No. 63 in Quantitative Applications in the Social Sciences. Newbury Park, CA: Sage Publications.

Ethridge, D., & McSweeney, M. (1971). Research in occupational therapy. Part III Research designs. *American Journal of Occupational Therapy, XXV*(1), 24–28.

Fetterman, D. (1989). *Ethnography: Step by step.* No. 17 in Applied Social Research Methods Series. Newbury Park, CA: Sage Publications.

Fielding, N. G., & Fielding, J. L. (1986). *Linking data.* No. 4 in Qualitative Research Methods Series. Newbury Park, CA: Sage Publications.

Fink, A., & Kosecoff, J. (1985). *How to conduct surveys.* Newbury Park, CA: Sage Publications.

Fowler, F. J., & Mangione, T. W. (1989). *Standardized survey interviewing: Minimizing interviewer-related error.* No. 18 in Applied Social Research Methods Series. Newbury Park, CA: Sage Publications.

Frey, J. H. (1989). *Survey research by telephone.* No. 150 in Sage Library of Social Research. Newbury Park, CA: Sage Publications.

Gladwin, C. H. (1989). *Ethnographic decision tree modeling.* No. 19 in Qualitative Research Methods Series. Newbury Park, CA: Sage Publications.

Hacker, B. (1980). Part I Single subject research strategies in occupational therapy. *American Journal of Occupational Therapy, 34*(2), 103–108.

Hacker, B. (1980). Part II Single subject research strategies in occupational therapy. *American Journal of Occupational Therapy, 34*(3), 169–175.

Kalton, G. (1983). *Introduction to survey sampling.* No. 35 in Quantitative Applications in the Social Sciences. Newbury Park, CA: Sage Publications.

Kielhofner, G., & Burke, J. P. (1977). Occupational therapy after 60 years: An account of changing identity and knowledge. *American Journal of Occupational Therapy, 31*(10), 675–689.

Kraemer, H., & Thiemann, S. (1987). *How many subjects? Statistical power analysis in research.* Newbury Park, CA: Sage Publications.

Krueger, R. A. (1988). *Focus groups: A practical guide for applied research.* Newbury Park, CA: Sage Publications. The design, conduct and interpretation of group interviews in small human service organizations.

Lehmkuhl, D. (1970). Research. Let's reduce the understanding gap. Part III Experimental design: What and why? *Physical Therapy, 50*(12), 1716–1720.

Marshall, C., & Rossman, G. B. (1989). *Designing qualitative research.* Newbury Park, CA: Sage Publications.

Schmeckebier, L. F., & Eastin, R. B. (1969). *Government publications and their use.* Washington, DC: Brookings Institution.

Spector, P. (1981). *Research designs*. No. 23 in Quantitative Applications in the Social Sciences Series. Newbury Park, CA: Sage Publications.

Webb, E. J., Campbell, D. T., Schwartz, R. D., & Sechrest, C. (1966). *Unobtrusive measures: Normative research in the social sciences*. Chicago, IL: Rand McNally and Company.

West, W. (1979). Historical perspectives. In *Occupational Therapy: 2001 AD* (pp. 9–17). Rockville, MD: American Occupational Therapy Association.

Yerxa, E. J. (1979). The philosophical base of occupational therapy. In *Occupational Therapy: 2001 AD* (pp. 26–30). Rockville, MD: American Occupational Therapy Association.

Yin, R. K. (1981a). The case study as a serious research strategy. *Knowledge: Creation, Diffusion, Utilization, 3*(September), 97–114.

Yin, R. K. (1981b). The case study crisis: Some answers. *Administrative Science Quarterly, 26*(March), 58–65.

Yin, R. K. (1989). *Case study research: Design and methods*. No. 5 in Applied Social Science Research Methods Series. Newbury Park, CA: Sage Publications.

CHAPTER

6

Establishing Boundaries for the Study

A research study needs to be given boundaries and to be put into a context for readers. They should be able to understand quickly where a study fits into the scheme of professional literature, should be made aware of any assumptions the author has made about the underlying principles of the study, should know if there are any overriding problems that are likely to influence the results or interpretation of the results, and should be able to find the meanings of all terms used if they are not obvious. This information will enable readers to understand the researcher's general intentions and to follow the researcher's train of thought.

DEFINING AND OPERATIONALIZING TERMS

Some of the terms in the study need to be defined, while others need to be operationalized. In both cases, the specific meanings of the terms in your study need to be made clear to the reader. First, the simple definitions.

People reading your study may come from a variety of professional backgrounds and may not be familiar with terms idiosyncratic to your discipline or specialty. Terms should be defined so that the reader will know their precise meaning in the context of the study. It is also important to define terms that are technical to your field or that have everyday language counterparts with which they might be confused, such as the word *grounding*, which has a meaning in ethnography that is quite different from its nautical or baseball meaning.

It is important to define terms that occur in the problem statement, purpose of the study, and research questions or hypotheses, because a misunderstanding here could be pivotal to the reader's grasp of the entire study. Definitions may come from dictionaries, medical textbooks, lists of synonyms, glossaries, and so on, and may range from the simple substitution of words to elaborate explanations requiring several paragraphs (see Box 6–A).

It should be noted that Ritter (in Box 6–A) used existing definitions from authorities and cited the authors. This is a useful and acceptable procedure for defining terms.

Operationalizing terms goes one step further than simply substituting one term for another. The purpose is to remove speculation and non-observable words from the definition so that their meaning for the particular study under review cannot be misinterpreted.

74

Box 6–A

For a study whose hypothesis was that regular aerobic exercise will improve the cardiovascular fitness of adults with developmental disabilities (Ritter, 1989), simple definitions were used for two relevant terms:

"Aerobic exercise—Exercise during which the energy needed is supplied by the aerobic metabolism. Slow, rhythmic movement of large body muscles. Aerobic exercise is required for sustained periods of physical work and vigorous athletic exercise (Cooper, 1968).

Developmental disabilities—Conditions due to congenital abnormality, trauma, deprivation, or diseases occurring up to the age of 22 years that interrupt or delay the sequence and rate of normal growth, development, and maturation (Massachusetts Developmental Disabilities Council, 1985)."

(p. 15)

The reason for this exercise is to make scientific communication clear so that studies can be accurately replicated. To achieve such clarity, concepts are defined in terms of the operations by which they are measured. Thus, time is measured in commonly identifiable quantities, such as minutes or days, and length is represented by feet or inches. The goal is for you to provide your readers with the type of information that will allow them to know what to do in order to experience that which is being defined.

Operational definitions can apply not only to measurable items, such as degrees of flexion, but also to concepts, such as independence or self-esteem. Operational definitions should always point to a specific example or referent. Chase (1966) listed four possible kinds of referent that could serve as the basis of operational definitions:

1. Material objects at given places and dates: This splint here; this patient with carpal tunnel syndrome; this rehabilitation hospital.
2. Collections of objects at given places and dates: The patients with cardiac conditions in Sunnyview Nursing Home on August 4, 1988.
3. Happenings at given places and dates: The passage of the Health Maintenance Organization legislation in Washington on July 29, 1986.
4. Processes verified scientifically: Normal body temperature is approximately 98.6°F.

Francis, Bork, and Carstens (1984) add a fifth referent:

5. The personal experience of a given individual as reported by that individual: Freud's Oedipus Complex as his way of experiencing and explaining certain behavior patterns. Descriptions of personal experience are valid representations of individual thought even if there is no corresponding external referent. Even Thomas Szasz's notion of "the myth of mental illness" can be operationally defined in terms of what Szasz thinks a person must know to understand that myth.

In Box 6–B, the first sentence would have been sufficient for a simple definition. However, Middlebrook wanted to operationalize the term *heart rate* in order to make it specific to her study, so she added the last two sentences to make it an operational definition. Boxes 6–C and 6–D contain examples of simple definitions and operational

---

Box 6–B

In Middlebrook's (1988) study titled *The effect of functional movement patterns on hemodynamic response in older individuals*, the definition of heart rate reads:

Heart Rate (HR): "The number of ventricular beats per minute" (Astrand & Rodahl, 1970; p. 122), resulting from contraction of the ventricles. This measurement was taken by counting the number of QRS complexes detected by the ARS beeper on the ECG monitor in a 15 second period, then multiplying by 4. It was recorded in beats per minute (bpm).

(p. 25)

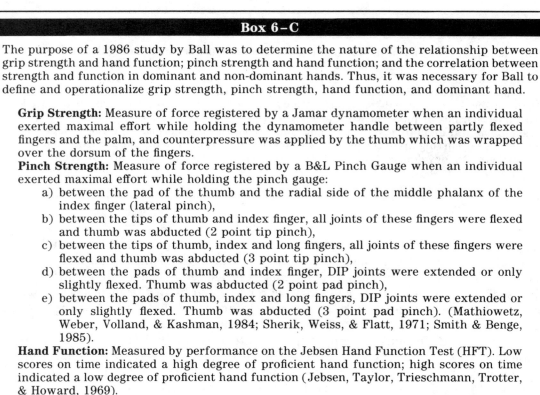

Box 6-C

The purpose of a 1986 study by Ball was to determine the nature of the relationship between grip strength and hand function; pinch strength and hand function; and the correlation between strength and function in dominant and non-dominant hands. Thus, it was necessary for Ball to define and operationalize grip strength, pinch strength, hand function, and dominant hand.

Grip Strength: Measure of force registered by a Jamar dynamometer when an individual exerted maximal effort while holding the dynamometer handle between partly flexed fingers and the palm, and counterpressure was applied by the thumb which was wrapped over the dorsum of the fingers.

Pinch Strength: Measure of force registered by a B&L Pinch Gauge when an individual exerted maximal effort while holding the pinch gauge:
  a) between the pad of the thumb and the radial side of the middle phalanx of the index finger (lateral pinch),
  b) between the tips of thumb and index finger, all joints of these fingers were flexed and thumb was abducted (2 point tip pinch),
  c) between the tips of thumb, index and long fingers, all joints of these fingers were flexed and thumb was abducted (3 point tip pinch),
  d) between the pads of thumb and index finger, DIP joints were extended or only slightly flexed. Thumb was abducted (2 point pad pinch),
  e) between the pads of thumb, index and long fingers, DIP joints were extended or only slightly flexed. Thumb was abducted (3 point pad pinch). (Mathiowetz, Weber, Volland, & Kashman, 1984; Sherik, Weiss, & Flatt, 1971; Smith & Benge, 1985).

Hand Function: Measured by performance on the Jebsen Hand Function Test (HFT). Low scores on time indicated a high degree of proficient hand function; high scores on time indicated a low degree of proficient hand function (Jebsen, Taylor, Trieschmann, Trotter, & Howard, 1969).

Dominant Hand: The dominant hand was the hand which the subject preferred most often in Annett's Hand Preference Questionnaire (Annett, 1970a).

(pp. 6-7)

definitions from two theses. It is worth taking time to define terms accurately and completely to prevent confusion later on.

ASSUMPTIONS

At this point, you need to think about assumptions you are making about the study and the premises upon which the study is being formulated. It is customary for researchers to examine their own assumptions carefully and to state them to the reader near the begin-

Box 6-D

The purpose of a 1989 study by Moore was to evaluate the effectiveness of an individualized guided visual imagery program for patients with psychosomatic, psychogenic, or chronic somatic disorders. He defined terms in the following manner:

"**Psychogenic Illnesses:** somatic illnesses created by the mind or mental state.
Psychosomatic Illnesses: somatic illnesses exacerbated by the mind or mental state.
Somatic Illnesses: states of illness that originate in the body secondary to trauma, disease process, or malfunction of one or more body systems.
Responses: monitored physiological states including electromyograph, galvanic skin response, heart rate, respiration rate, peripheral thermal reading, amount of medication.
Individualized, guided visual imagery: images created by the therapist or the patient that use one or more of the five senses to create a temporarily believable illusion, that is specifically designed to meet the needs of the patient as dictated by their individual personality, preferences, and language format."

(pp. 7-8)

ning of the study. If this is done, readers need not agree with the researcher's assumptions but are able to follow the logic of propositions and to understand why the specific study approach was taken.

Assumptions are underlying principles that the researcher believes or accepts but that are difficult to prove in any concrete way. They are frequently untested and untestable hypotheses, basic values, or views about the world. They include such values as the notion that people are basically good or that people want to function independently in their day-to-day activities. These ideas would be very difficult to prove with the population at large or even with a small research group.

Two kinds of assumptions should be examined: First, assumptions about the ideological principles upon which the study is based and, second, assumptions that are made concerning the procedures used in the study. We all adhere to certain ingrained principles that will affect the way we look at situations and therefore the way we design research studies.

For example, in following their ideological principles, a client-centered researcher and a financially oriented researcher might approach the previously mentioned study about the use of aerobic exercise with developmentally delayed adults (Ritter, 1989) from quite different viewpoints. The client-centered researcher might hold the assumption that developmentally delayed adults deserve the fun and sense of well-being often promoted by aerobic exercise and would investigate ways of bringing such exercise to those residing in sheltered living situations with this in mind. The money-conscious administrative researcher might feel that aerobic exercise contributes to physical health and that regular participation may reduce the cost of medical care for developmentally delayed adults who are supported financially by the state.

The two researchers are likely to adopt different study methods in approaching the benefits of bringing aerobic exercise to developmentally delayed adults who receive state support. The first researcher would probably investigate the results of the exercise on the well-being and enjoyment level of subjects, while the second might investigate the results of the exercise on the health status and resulting health care costs of the subjects.

The second type of assumption relates to the procedures used during the research study. Usually these pertain to the instruments used and the willingness of subjects to participate in the study. For instance, researchers often are obliged to assume that the measuring instrument being used is valid and reliable because, in human subject research anyway, it is often difficult to prove validity and reliability conclusively. The most notoriously unreliable instruments are interviews and questionnaires, yet it is sometimes impossible to conduct a study without them. Box 6–E illustrates how one author clearly states the major assumption of her study.

There are other basic assumptions associated with the use of measuring instruments, such as assuming that the subjects will answer questions honestly or that they will respond to tests of skill to the best of their ability. In making procedural assumptions, the researcher must try to think in advance of all eventualities and control the research design as much as possible. For example, in some studies where performance is being measured on a test of skill, it is imperative for the study that subjects try as hard as they can on the test. To ensure this, some researchers have devised reward systems to compensate subjects according to their motivation level. When these sorts of strategies are used, assumptions

---

Box 6–E

The objective of Schwartzberg's study (1982) was to learn, from the perspective of the psychiatric patient, what facilitates or blocks occupational performance. Twenty-four adult patients from a psychiatric unit were interviewed with a set of open-ended questions. Their answers were thematically analyzed, leading to inferences about what these patients felt facilitated or blocked their occupational performance. Schwartzberg's assumption was as follows:

> The study was based on the assumption that listening to and analyzing patients' reports is a profitable way to understand factors relevant to function and dysfunction in their occupational performance.

(p. 3)

need to be made less frequently and only for those items beyond the researcher's control and ingenuity.

It can be seen that making your assumptions known in the early stages of describing a study is most important so that readers know where you stand on issues related to the research and where they should keep a critical eye on procedures.

SCOPE OF THE STUDY

In the significance section you developed after reading Chapter 3, you showed why your study, among all possible studies that the problem might generate, was worth undertaking. Any problem can be approached from different angles, yet the researcher has selected a specific angle or approach. Therefore, it is necessary to explain that approach to the reader. This is known as *defining the study's scope*. It is insufficient to merely state, "This is the approach I am taking." A rationale must be provided—a set of constructs and principles that will guide the reader to a clear and focused understanding of the researcher's frame of reference. This set of guiding constructs and principles is called the conceptual framework of the study and serves as a structure for the scope.

For example, in King's work (1974) with chronic schizophrenic patients, she made it clear to readers that she was taking the guiding constructs and principles of A. Jean Ayres's theories on sensory integration and adapting them for use with a new client population. She explained the portion of Ayres's theory she was using, defined her research population precisely, and stated why she thought the particular frame of reference described was an appropriate approach to use. King's article is an excellent example of documentation for a research project's scope.

The scope section may not always be as elaborately and meticulously presented as King's, however. She chose to spend so much time on this point because she was presenting a new treatment choice for a particular client population. Her study encompassed the crucial underlying constructs and principles that the reader needed to understand and accept in order for the ensuing research to be logical and meaningful. In studies where the point of the study is not contingent on the scope or conceptual framework chosen, it is customary to merely set the stage for the reader with a paragraph on the subject (see Box 6-F).

The conceptual framework focuses the study and narrows it to just one of myriad possibilities. It tells the reader what that focus is, what will be covered in the project, and what will not be included. For instance, if a sensory integrative approach is to be taken in a study, it would not be reasonable to expect the researcher to cover the possibilities of what might happen to subjects if a behavioral approach had been used.

Informing the reader of the conceptual framework and therefore the scope of the project puts the study in a context, both in the literature and in the work that was previously accomplished using that framework. In this way, it was immediately apparent

---

Box 6-F

Middlebrook's (1988) study of the effect of functional movement patterns on hemodynamic responses in older individuals contains a good example of a brief description of the conceptual framework of her study, which in this case was a previously documented frame of reference.

This investigation was based on the biomechanical frame of reference, which, according to Trombley (1983), "deals with increasing strength, endurance, and range of joint motion in patients who have an intact central nervous system but who have dysfunction in the peripheral nervous system or the musculoskeletal, integumentary, or cardio-pulmonary systems" (pp. 1-2). In the present investigation, the endurance of subjects performing an upper extremity activity was studied through monitoring. . . .

(pp. 27-28)

to readers that King's work was adding to the body of knowledge about sensory integrative techniques as a form of treatment. Knowledgeable readers on that topic knew that a new group of patients was being added to those who currently benefit from sensory integrative treatment.

Besides setting the study in a context for the reader, defining the scope of the study often helps investigators put limits on their own work. They can feel comfortable stating what is and what is not within the scope of their studies. In this way, the scope acts as a delimiting factor, marking the boundaries of material that should be covered.

LIMITATIONS OF THE STUDY

The limitations section of the study should include the conceptual and methodological shortcomings that cannot be overcome in the study design. They may include such things as not being able to randomly select the subjects, not being able to include a control group, or not having a standardized instrument available to measure variables. There may be methodological problems that cannot be overcome, such as not having access to a mailing list of exactly the people you want to poll in an attitude survey, and having to make do with an overinclusive or underinclusive list (see Box 6–G). Or there may be conceptual limitations, such as an underlying principle of the study not being widely accepted outside the professional specialty of the researcher.

Naturally, listing the limitations of a study does not excuse the researcher from making all possible attempts to overcome the problems. But after considering all possible improvements, pointing out the remaining limitations shows that you are aware of them and will consider them in discussing the results.

SUBJECTS

At this point, a word is in order about the subjects in your research project. Because most projects involve the examination of evidence that bears upon the hypotheses, the sources for that evidence—the subjects—need to be clearly identified. Studies of ongoing programs and historical studies will rely heavily on documents, records, and verbal reports as evidence, while experimental research investigating such things as efficacy of treatment will be more apt to use individuals to supply the evidence. Thus, subjects may be people, written records, tape recordings, observations, or verbal reports.

The criteria are established ahead of subject selection to ensure that subjects with appropriate attributes make up the sample. Criteria are determined from the theoretical underpinnings of the study, as determined from the literature review (see Box 6–H).

When subjects are described, a clear distinction between the population and the sample

---

Box 6–G

In Nelson's study of self-esteem and professionalism in female occupational therapists (1989), limitations are identified as follows:

> Since the sample size was not large, and the cross-section of respondents not wide, it was impossible to make generalizations about the entire population of occupational therapists. Because this was a case study of occupational therapists in Massachusetts, it was difficult to draw conclusions about occupational therapists at large. Another limitation was that the variables chosen for study (self-esteem and professionalism) are only contributing factors to some of the larger problems of the profession outlined here. That is, they comprise a small piece of the larger puzzle.

(pp. 5–6)

Box 6-H

In designing an alternative splint for clients with carpal tunnel syndrome (CTS), Mawn (1990) wanted to test the splint on subjects who had not used a splint previously and had not been operated on for CTS prior to the study. This was to allow for a controlled study, comparing subjects using the new splint to a control group using prior methods of treatment. Additionally, Mawn wanted subjects of both sexes who were employed and taking sick leave because of CTS symptoms to determine if they could return to work using the new splint sooner than those in the control group. Thus, the population criteria were: Men and women with CTS, who had not received a splint or had an operation, and who were on sick leave from their jobs.

---

is necessary. The population is the total group, set of events, or theoretical constructs to which your hypotheses apply. The criteria or characteristics of these people/items in the population must be clearly defined. A sample is a smaller subset of the population that has been selected for study in your particular project. The method of selection should be such that the sample represents the population as closely as possible. The process of random, selection (described in Chapter 4) is often used.

Later, when the sample has been selected, their demographic data will be collected and included in the description of the study results. For the Mawn study (in Box 6-H), this might include such information as the subjects' type of employment, how long they have been absent from their jobs, and any previous treatment they have received for carpal tunnel syndrome. In summary, the population parameters and criteria are established before subject selection according to indicators from the literature, while information about the sample subjects is described later, after the sample has been selected.

Selection criteria are established as the assumptions and theoretical base of the study unfold. Criteria are dictated by the theory behind why the researcher feels the intervention will be helpful (e.g., King's theory, based on many years' observations, that only schizophrenic patients of the non-paranoid type can be expected to benefit from sensory-integrative treatment).

Examples of populations and samples from actual studies may be found in Boxes 6-I, 6-J, and 6-K. These examples all provide clear selection criteria for the individuals or written records in the study populations and samples. Unfortunately, none of these researchers was able to randomly select their sample subjects. As we have seen in the previous discussion of random selection, this process is highly desirable but difficult to achieve in reality.

Box 6-I

Clifford and Bundy (1989) administered the Preschool Play Scale and Preschool Play Materials Preference Inventory to 66 preschool-age boys, in order to examine whether or not play preference and play performance of boys with sensory-integrative dysfunction were different from the preferences of normal boys in this age group. The *population* under study were all preschool-age boys in Massachusetts participating in day-care centers or day camps. The *subjects*, who were not randomly selected, consisted of

> sixty-six 4-, 5-, and 6-year-old boys, divided into two groups matched in age, verbal intelligence (single word receptive vocabulary), and socioeconomic status. Group 1 consisted of 35 normal boys recruited from day-care centers and a day camp in the Boston area. Group 2 consisted of 31 boys diagnosed by an experienced occupational therapist with training in SI theory and evaluation as having SI dysfunction. . . . Group 2 subjects were recruited from three occupational therapy private practices, an occupational therapy teaching clinic, and two children's hospitals, all in Massachusetts.

(pp. 205-206)

Box 6–J

In Moore's study (1989) investigating whether guided visual imagery was a viable modality for occupational therapists, a retrospective chart review was used as the research method. In this instance, the *population* consisted of all the charts of patients seen at a hospital in Massachusetts during a specific 2-year period. The *subjects* were the charts of those patients seen by one occupational therapist who were diagnosed with psychogenic, psychosomatic, or chronic somatic disorders, and who had received guided visual imagery as a treatment modality.

STUMBLING BLOCKS

ASSUMPTIONS

People often make the mistake of including in the assumptions section those notions they hold about the study that can be proved—in other words, those ideas that are referenced in scientific literature. As soon as ideas are "proved" scientifically, they need no longer be presented as assumptions but rather should be presented in the literature review section as part of the reason for conducting the study in a certain manner. Only beliefs that are difficult to prove in any concrete way—beliefs that are untested or untestable hypotheses, basic values, or views about the world—should be included in the assumptions section.

SCOPE

The distinction between the assumptions underlying a research project and the scope of the project is sometimes blurred. Remember that assumptions are individual and often unrelated beliefs about the nature of the topic. The scope, on the other hand, presents an encompassing conceptual framework in which to place the whole study. This frame of reference will color all aspects of the research and will provide a backdrop against which the reader may view the entire study.

LIMITATIONS

I advise students not to give litanies of limitations for their studies. After a while, it begins to look as if the study never should have been attempted when, in fact, the study may have proved quite useful in advancing an area of knowledge. There is a middle ground to be achieved between (1) listing every conceivable problem and quirk in a study and (2) being fair with the reader and presenting those things that could truly bias the results. Knowledgeable readers will pick up obvious limitations but will respect an author who acknowledges problems and considers them in the interpretation of the findings.

Box 6–K

In her 1988 study Middlebrook used all the men and women in Massachusetts between the ages of 60 and 79 as her *population*. Her *subjects* were 23 women and 7 men who volunteered to participate and who were "without a history of cardiovascular disease, systemic hypertension (blood pressure greater than 150/90 mm/Hg), chronic obstructive pulmonary disease . . . , or cerebrovascular accident. The medical histories of the subjects were determined by self-report."
(p. 27)

WORKSHEETS

DEFINITION OF TERMS

Have someone outside your discipline review the problem statement, purpose of the study, and research questions or hypotheses. Have the person point out words or phrases he or she does not understand.

List here words you feel need either a simple definition or an operational definition:

Problem statement words:
Definition   Operational definition

Words from the purpose of the study:
Definition   Operational definition

Hypothesis words:
Definition   Operational definition

Go through the list and decide for each word if the definition should come from a dictionary, glossary, textbook, professional authority/group, etc.

Write a definition for each word in the:

Problem statement:

Purpose:

Hypothesis:

ASSUMPTIONS

Read through the problem statement, the background, the purpose of the study, and the significance. As you read, see if you have made any assumptions about your population, the environment in which it functions, or the intervention being proposed that need to be presented to the reader.

Assumption 1:

Assumption 2:

Assumption 3:

SCOPE OF THE STUDY

What is the underlying framework or scope for your study? Are you following an accepted theoretical frame of reference, such as a behavioral or developmental approach or a biomechanical model? State your conceptual framework here:

Write two or three paragraphs describing why you are approaching the study from this perspective and how the chosen conceptual framework will shape the study.

LIMITATIONS

Reread the early sections of your study looking for conceptual limitations. List them here.

Reread the methodology section of your study looking for procedural limitations. List them here:

SUBJECT SELECTION

Will the subjects for your study be clients, patients, written records, tape recordings, verbal reports, observations, or other?

Define the selection criteria for the population (from whom your sample will be chosen):

Examples:
- All of the written records, photographs, and tape-recorded interviews relating to the founding of the American Physical Therapy Association.
- All of the occupational therapists working in psychiatric hospitals in Massachusetts.

Add relevant criteria to the description of the population based on the literature review and the design of the study.

Example:
- Occupational therapists currently working in Massachusetts state-supported psychiatric hospitals who are working with schizophrenic patients.

Do you know the approximate number in the population?

How will the sample be selected from the population?

_____ Random selection   _____ Other

Describe:

How many will the sample comprise?

Will the sample be divided into experimental and control groups?

How will group assignment be made?

_____ Random assignment   _____ Other

Describe:

REFERENCES

Ball, J. H. (1986). *Pinch and grip strength related to performance on the Jebsen Hand Function Test*. Unpublished master's thesis, Tufts University, Medford, MA.

Chase, S. (1966). *The tyranny of words*. New York: Harcourt, Brace & World.

Clifford, J., & Bundy, A. (1989). Play preference and play performance in normal boys and boys with sensory integrative dysfunction. *The Occupational Therapy Journal of Research, 9*(4), 202–217.

Francis, J., Bork, C., & Carstens, S. (1984). *The proposal cookbook: A step by step guide to dissertation and thesis proposal writing*. Naples, FL: Action Research Associates.

King, L. J. (1974). A sensory-integrative approach to schizophrenia. *American Journal of Occupational Therapy, 28*(9), 529–536.

Mawn, M. (1990). *The dorsal-ulnar splint as a treatment for carpal tunnel syndrome: A case study*. Unpublished master's thesis, Tufts University, Medford, MA.

Middlebrook, J. A. (1988). *The effect of functional movement patterns on hemodynamic responses in older individuals*. Unpublished master's thesis, Tufts University, Medford, MA.

Moore, D. A. (1989). *Guided visual imagery as an occupational therapy modality*. Unpublished master's thesis, Tufts University, Medford, MA.

Nelson, B. J. (1989). *Self-esteem and professionalism in female occupational therapists*. Unpublished master's thesis, Tufts University, Medford, MA.

Ritter, J. (1989). *Aerobic exercise with adults with developmental disabilities*. Unpublished master's thesis, Tufts University, Medford, MA.

Schwartzberg, S. L. (1982). Motivation for activities of daily living: A study of selected psychiatric patients' self-reports. *Occupational Therapy in Mental Health, 2*(3), 1–26.

ADDITIONAL READING

Berger, R. M., & Patchner, M. A. (1988). *Planning for research: A guide for the helping professions*. No. 50 in the Sage Human Services Guides Series. Newbury Park, CA: Sage Publications.

Stein, F. (1989). Chapter 6: Research Design. In *Anatomy of clinical research: An introduction to scientific inquiry in medicine, rehabilitation and related health professions* (pp. 165–175). Thorofare, NJ: Slack, Inc.

Collecting and Analyzing Qualitative Data

Now that you have decided upon a method to use to carry out your study, you must decide upon ways to collect and analyze the data. Your research may have generated either quantitative or qualitative data. Quantitative data result from variables that can be enumerated in some way so as to be tabulated and subjected to statistical procedures. The analysis of quantitative data will be discussed in Chapter 8. Qualitative data, on the other hand, are non-numerical in nature and cannot be measured directly (e.g., attitudes, values, degree of participation, facial expressions, and adjectives describing feelings). When numbers or units are assigned to components of such variables (known as attributes), statistical analysis can be made using appropriate statistical procedures. These will be discussed in Chapter 8, "Analyzing Quantitative Data." When no such assignment of a numerical value is given to the attribute, other methods of data analysis must be used. These methods will be addressed in this chapter.

DATA COLLECTION METHODS

Sometimes the research method will dictate data collection methods; for example, ethnographic research methodology implies the use of field data collection techniques such as observation and interviews, while survey research will always involve either interviews (by telephone or in person) or written questionnaires. However, in using other research methods, data collection techniques are less clear and the investigator often has a wide array of choices.

To illuminate the choices, let us categorize data collection possibilities and discuss each of them. Methods may be conveniently grouped as follows:

1. Observation
2. Interview
3. Questionnaire
4. Record review
5. Hardware instrumentation
6. Tests, measures, and inventories

OBSERVATION

This data collection technique may be used in any of the research designs—experimental, quasi-experimental, and non-experimental—and is commonly used in conjunction with other techniques. Observations may be made of human subjects, of videotape recordings of subjects or events, of non-human items such as pieces of equipment, or of scores on written protocols or ratings.

Rather than being asked to observe and record subjective items such as "dependence" or "enjoyment," observers should be given objective criteria believed to represent those subjective items. For example, "dependence" in a given study may be represented by the number of times a subject asks for assistance, and "enjoyment" may be represented by the number of smiles, the number of laughs, or the number of verbal statements that would indicate happiness. Observers should be provided with a protocol defining the items to be observed and a method for recording those items, such as noting any occurrence, frequency of occurrence, or length of time between occurrences.

Further, observers should be trained in making their observations. Videotapes can be useful for training purposes. The observer rates the tapes, and the researcher checks the ratings until he or she is satisfied that the observer is making correct and reliable ratings. If there is more than one observer or rater, the researcher will probably want to use a technique called interrater reliability, which means the raters are not only checked individually but are also checked against one another. This reliability check is carried out until all raters score similarly and the researcher has confidence, borne out by statistics, that they will rate consistently well.

The importance of raters' impartiality, so as to protect the internal validity of the study, cannot be stressed enough. This issue is addressed more fully in the "Stumbling Blocks" section at the end of this chapter.

INTERVIEW

The interview is one of the methods used to gather data in survey and ethnographic research and may be conducted face to face or by telephone. Interviews conducted face to face are more intimate, allowing the interviewer to interact directly and develop rapport with the interviewee. This may be important if sensitive issues are being explored; the interviewee can be put at ease, reassured, and encouraged to give candid answers. Additionally, the interviewer has a chance to "read" the non-verbal cues given by the interviewee, which may indicate confusion or lack of understanding, so that a question can be rephrased. Non-verbal information may also be an important part of understanding the full response to the question.

The disadvantage of face-to-face interviews is the amount of effort required to set up the interview—contacting subjects, arranging mutually convenient times and places, traveling, setting up rooms. Telephone interviewing cuts down on travel time and arrangements are easier to make, but the personal contact and the chance to observe non-verbal cues are lost. Also, it is easier for a subject to refuse an interview on the telephone.

The interview format may be structured or unstructured, sometimes referred to as formal or informal. In structured interviews, the same questions are always asked, and they are asked in the same order. Although this format may appear stilted and formal, it does mean that the answers will be easier to compare from one subject to another and that the information from all subjects will be consistent.

In unstructured interviews, the interviewer must be trained to know what is essential information for the research and must be entirely familiar with the questions before starting the interview. Although informal interviewing is often more comfortable for the interviewee and is useful in obtaining a great deal of detailed information, the volume of material can be most difficult to organize and analyze, and often is not comparable from one subject to the next. Accordingly, one cannot compare across subjects easily or compile frequencies and percentages easily. If the researcher is carrying out survey research, the

Box 7-A

Converse and Presser (1986) state:

"Forbid" and "allow" . . . are logical opposites, and thus substituting one for the other in the question "Do you think the United States should [allow/forbid] public speeches against democracy?" might easily be assumed to have no effect. Yet it turns out that many more people are willing to "not allow" such speeches than are willing to "forbid" them. (p. 41)

implication is that he or she will discover something about a whole group of people and will want similar information from each person to compare and contrast.

When should you use a structured as opposed to an unstructured interview? It depends on the purpose of the data collection and what you want to achieve. You may use unstructured interviews in a pilot study, to set the parameters of the study. Once the issues have been clarified, you may move to a structured interview for the formal study.

In using unstructured interviews, the researcher is often "fishing," not wanting to be boxed in by specific formal questions. However, there is the danger of getting too far off track and of losing the original sense of purpose for the study. Results from the procedure can be amorphous because the material differs from subject to subject, and it can be difficult to know what to do with it all. Nevertheless, one can get an in-depth feel for that individual subject or topic, and in this way the unstructured interview can be useful as a tool in pilot studies. Unstructured interviews may also be beneficial when questioning subjects about sensitive or awkward topics. The skillful interviewer can reword or reorder questions and introduce additional questions in order to put the subject at ease and to move at each subject's own pace.

Formal interviews, on the other hand, are probably best used by the inexperienced interviewer and the beginning researcher. The data will be more easily tabulated and analyzed, and interpretations are more likely to be accurate and meaningful.

In deciding on the wording of questions, prime consideration should be given to the language style and idiom used by subjects, which may well be different from that used by the researcher. During the interview, do not try to use the respondent's accent, but in all question development, try to use words and language similar to those used by the subjects. It is especially important not to use words foreign to respondents, such as medical terms (e.g., use *stroke* rather than *cerebrovascular accident*). Remove highly charged words from the interview and substitute more moderate words with the same meaning (see Box 7-A).

One of the problems with data obtained from interviews is that it is difficult to know if subjects are telling the truth or if they are trying to impress the interviewer by saying what they think the interviewer wants to hear. They may also be embarrassed or ashamed to tell the truth on sensitive issues. Experienced interviewers can gain skill in reading non-verbal cues to determine the degree of truthfulness in answers.

There is a great deal to be learned about the construction of individual questions and the interview as a whole. Since most of this information pertains to questionnaires as well as interviews, it will be discussed in the following section on questionnaires.

QUESTIONNAIRE

There are three ways to distribute written questionnaires. They may be mailed to respondents or given to respondents personally with instructions to mail them back to the researcher, or respondents may complete the questionnaire in the presence of the researcher. If questionnaires have been mailed or left for subjects to complete and return, there are special considerations. First, the questions must be very clear and unambiguous because the researcher will not be present to answer inquiries. This is of particular concern because if a question has been misinterpreted and answered incorrectly, the whole questionnaire must be discarded unless special statistical procedures are followed in analyzing results.

Another big concern researchers have regarding mailed questionnaires is whether there will be a sufficient response rate to justify the study. A reasonable response rate to expect if you are mailing to a group known to have an interest in the topic under study is about 30 percent. But there are ways to improve a response rate. The survey must be attractive and pleasing so that recipients will not discard it without reading the cover letter and initial instructions. The cover letter must be written so as to catch and hold the recipients' attention, and the topic must interest them sufficiently that they will want to answer the questions.

Questionnaires must be short enough that subjects will finish them but long enough to obtain the required information. There is a great deal written on the topic of how long questionnaires should be (Fink & Kosecoff, 1985). Self-administered questionnaires are generally limited to 30 minutes, while face-to-face interviews can continue for more than an hour (see Boxes 7–B and 7–C). One good rule of thumb is to view your questionnaire as objectively as you can and to ask yourself if you would stick with it and answer all the questions if it came to you in the mail.

Make sure that the cover letter tells the recipients why they should be interested in the study and what benefits they can expect from participating (even if it is only that they will be assisting a therapy student to complete her or his thesis and will thereby be indirectly helping to add one more person to the pool of working therapists). Capture their interest in the project by telling what you hope to achieve as a result of the study.

Always give a deadline for returning the questionnaire — approximately 2 weeks after it has been received. Research shows that recipients rarely return questionnaires after 2 weeks. Unless returns are confidential, keep a master list of those to whom you have mailed and check off their returns. If you have not heard from them in 2 weeks, send them a reminder postcard.

Always enclose a stamped, addressed envelope. This will increase the response rate a good deal. Recipients will generally not make the required effort to find an envelope and find your address on the cover letter (which has often been destroyed), and they may resent having to pay postage for your research project.

When constructing questions for questionnaires and interviews, two types of questions — closed-ended and open-ended — may be used. Closed-ended questions are those that require only a simple answer, usually yes or no or a check mark against a series of options, while open-ended questions are those that respondents can answer in as many words as they please.

Open-ended questions are most useful in dealing with complicated information when slight differences of opinion are important to know. Second, they provide a good way to elaborate on a closed-ended question, such as:

Do you teach clinical reasoning skills to your therapy students? Yes _____ No _____

If yes, please explain how and at what point in the curriculum:

Third, open-ended questions may be used as a way of finding out which issue in a series of closed-ended questions is the most important or most relevant to the respondent. For example, a series of specific questions about specialty certification may be followed by the question "What is your opinion of specialty certification?" This technique is useful in

Box 7–B

A local health clinic is concerned that it continue to meet the needs of a changing community. In recent years, many more of its patients are older than 65 years of age, and a substantial percentage speak English as a second language. A bilingual volunteer will be devoting two mornings a week for 8 weeks to a 45-minute face-to-face interview with users of the clinic. A 50-item survey form has been designed for the purpose.

Box 7-C

The neighborhood clinic is also concerned that its services be appropriate for a population that is getting older, many of whom prefer not to speak English. The city has decided to sponsor a survey of its clinic patients' needs. To minimize the amount of time that staff and patients will have to spend on the survey, a 10-minute, 6-item self-administered questionnaire is prepared. To facilitate the survey's efficiency, questionnaires are left at the receptionist's desk.

that it often makes respondents feel better after having been "boxed in" for possible answers—they can now say what they want to say. You might not use the open-ended piece of information in tabulating results, but it keeps the respondents interested and involved, and increases their chances of completing the survey.

Open-ended questions are useful in allowing respondents to answer in any style and manner they wish, without giving them suggestions. This reduces the chance of their giving what they perceive as socially acceptable answers. Similarly, questions that may be viewed as sensitive or threatening are usually best handled as open-ended questions and may be more honestly answered on an anonymous questionnaire than in a personal interview.

Respondents are often more willing to go quickly through a questionnaire composed of closed-ended questions rather than write several sentences that they have to think about and compose. However, the closed-ended responses may not satisfy the investigator who would prefer more detailed and personal responses. There is a trade-off here and the choice must be made by the researcher (see Box 7-D).

In closed-ended questions, response formats should be mutually exclusive and where ratings are required, there should be a wide array of choices. In the yes/no answer, there are differing opinions about whether to include the "don't know" option. Some people feel it gives respondents an easy way out and would rather force them into a positive or negative answer, while others feel it is only fair and that respondents deserve that option (see Box 7-E).

There are several ways in which test takers may be asked to respond to test items. As well as the simple yes/no response, respondents may be asked to fill in the blank or to choose a relevant response from a list. Yet other questions rely on some sort of rating scale, the best known being the semantic differential and the Likert rating scale. The semantic differential, developed by Charles Osgood (Osgood, Suci, & Tannenbaum, 1957), is used as a measure of affective meaning. Respondents are given a domain of concern and are asked to rate their affective responses about that domain on a list of bipolar scales. These are 7-point scales with opposing adjectives at the two extremes. Generally, there are three dimensions into which these adjective pairs can be categorized—the evaluative dimension (good/bad), the potency dimension (strong/weak), and the activity dimension (fast/slow). Box 7-F shows one use of the semantic differential.

In the Likert scale (Likert, 1932), a statement is given to respondents to indicate the

Box 7-D

"In an open versus closed question experiment, people were asked what they thought was the most important problem facing the nation (Schuman & Presser, 1981). As the survey began, the U.S. was hit with an unexpected natural-gas shortage. This was reflected on the open version, where 22% said the "energy shortage" was the most important problem. On the closed version, designed without knowledge of the energy problem, there was hardly a trace of concern about the shortage, over 99% choosing one of the five offered alternatives. . . . Thus, when not enough is known to write appropriate response categories, open ended questions are to be preferred."
(Converse & Presser, 1986, p. 34)

Box 7-E

"The problem [addressed in the question] is intensified by the standard survey practice of not including "don't know" or "no opinion" as a response option mentioned in the question. Experimental research shows that many more people will say "don't know" when that alternative is explicitly offered than when it is not. Such filtering for no opinion generally affects from about an eighth to a third of those interviewed."
(Converse & Presser, 1986, p. 35)

---

domain of concern, and the respondents are asked to indicate their level of agreement with that statement on a 5-point or 7-point scale. The 5-point scale is typically worded as follows: "Strongly agree, Agree, Neutral, Disagree, Strongly disagree." The 7-point scale would add "Very strongly agree" and "Very strongly disagree" at either end.

Incomplete sentences are sometimes used to find out such things as opinions, attitudes, knowledge, styles of behavior, or personality traits. A phrase is provided to indicate the domain of concern, and the respondent is asked to complete the sentence. For example, "My opinion about placing mentally retarded persons in group homes is. . . ."

Multiple-choice items can be used to elicit opinions or attitudes from respondents. A statement is provided, sometimes in question form, and respondents are asked to select the item from the list that most reflects their opinion, attitude, or even a likely action, such as is shown in Box 7-G.

In rank-ordering items, a list of items is provided and respondents are asked to place a number beside each, indicating their order of importance. Sometimes only the first two or three items of importance are asked for, and sometimes the whole list must be prioritized. It should be remembered that most people find it difficult to prioritize more than about 10 items.

Box 7-F

Henry, Nelson and Duncombe (1984) used the semantic differential to elicit subjects' responses on how they felt about themselves following a choice/no choice situation in an activity group, on three affective factors: evaluation, power, and activity. They used Osgood's short-form semantic differential where subjects were asked to assign a rating on a 7-point scale for each of 12 scales, 4 scales being identified with each factor. The actual scale looked like this:

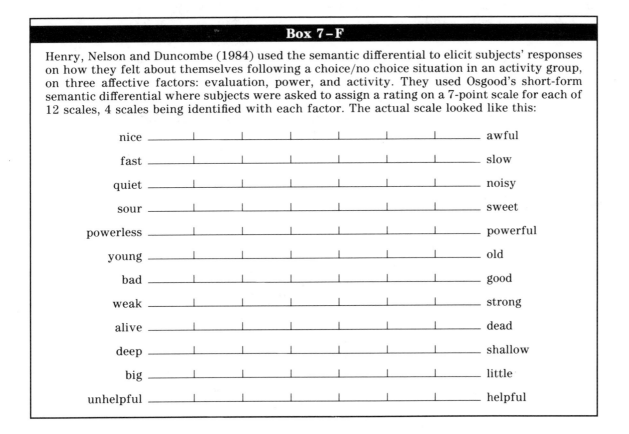

Box 7-G

Stein (1989) gives the example of a researcher surveying a group of post–myocardial-infarction patients on their attitudes toward their disability. This multiple-choice question might be found on the survey:

If I had a severe pain in my chest I would first do the following:
(a) Call my private physician
(b) Call an ambulance
(c) Call the emergency rescue unit of the police
(d) Lie down and rest
(e) Other, please specify: _____

(p. 119)

The questions should be sequenced so that they follow one another in a logical order. First, draw subjects into the interview and gain their interest with broad, general questions. Avoid sensitive questions until the respondent is comfortable and, in the case of a face-to-face interview, until rapport has been established.

It is a good idea not to give too many questions that require a simple yes or no or too many requiring a rating at different levels (such as "Rate on a scale of 1 to 5") in a sequence, because respondents lose interest and concentration after a while and answer without giving the questions much thought. Break up these questions with ones written in a different format.

Often researchers add a general open-ended question at the end of a questionnaire, designed to give the respondents an opportunity to add any information they did not have a chance to include during the process. On mailed questionnaires, it is quite common for respondents to write notes to the investigator, explaining things they think are unclear or adding items they feel are relevant. The final general question gives respondents a legitimate place to do this.

If you are planning to use the survey method in your research project, you are strongly advised to read one of the excellent books written about this specialized topic. Several such books are listed in the Additional Reading list at the end of this chapter.

RECORD REVIEW

Review of written records may be a means of data gathering in many types of research, including experimental, ethnographic, historical, and case study designs. In some types of research, such as the historical type, reviewing records and archival material may be the sole means of gathering data, while in others it is only one method.

Records reviewed may include patients' medical records, minutes of meetings and case conferences, letters, speeches, articles, books, diaries, photographs, and illustrations; physical materials such as equipment, artifacts, and clothing; or mechanical materials such as audio and video recordings or films.

Traditionally, records used as research data are divided into primary and secondary sources. Primary sources are firsthand accounts about the subject under review, such as autobiographies or eyewitness accounts, while secondary sources are accounts written about the subject by others but not based on personal experience (such as medical records). Investigators should try to verify both the truth about the writing of the documents (did this person actually write it?), as well as the truth about the content of the documents (did this actually happen?).

In summarizing and interpreting the data gathered, the researcher must use logical analysis and try to be as objective as possible. When examination of records is the only form of data gathering used in a study, the researcher cannot confirm that one event in the past caused another but must make assumptions or inferences that assign causality to historical events. The more information uncovered about an event, the more likely the cause of the event will become known. Investigators must be careful to restrict interpretations about causes and generalizability to the evidence gathered.

HARDWARE INSTRUMENTATION

Many studies performed by therapists employ physical measures of such functions as joint range, muscle strength, or galvanic skin response. Physical, mechanical instruments that provide a valid and reliable measurement are usually more desirable, in research terms, than the subjective feedback given by subjects. Before relying on a piece of equipment as a measuring instrument in a research study, however, the therapist should make sure that it really is reliable and valid. The use of equipment for measuring is also desirable in research because it provides a simple method for operationally defining independent variables (see Box 7–H).

In these days of sophisticated equipment in the medical arena, there are many choices available for measuring independent variables. Therapists use such instruments as cable tensiometers, spirometers, electroencephalographs, and goniometers, which are commonly referred to as hardware. In his book *Elements of Research in Physical Therapy*, Currier (1984) describes the use of scientific hardware, considerations of instrumentation such as manufacturers and specifications, and areas of research interests and the associated hardware used to measure relevant physiological responses. A list of publications that will assist the researcher in identifying and locating hardware is included in Appendix D.

Unfortunately, there are many variables that cannot be measured using hardware, and other means must be found to define and quantify them. These other means are generally written tests and measures, which will be discussed in the next section.

TESTS, MEASURES, AND INVENTORIES

A great deal of research data used by health professionals is gathered on written tests, measures, and inventories. Variables that may be measured by these written means include psychological factors, intelligence, perceptual motor skills, child development stages, prevocational skills, vocational interests, personality factors, attitudes and values. A list of the major suppliers of tests is given in Appendix E.

Some of the better-known tests have been gathered and critiqued in such bibliographic texts as Hemphill's book (1982) on tests used in the practice of occupational therapy in mental health, and two collections of tests and measures used for psychological assessment (Chun, Cobb, & French, 1985) and social psychological attitudes (Robinson & Shriver, 1985). Perhaps the best-known and most comprehensive books on the subject are Buros's *Tests in Print II: An Index to Tests, Test Reviews, and the Literature on Specific Tests* (1975), which lists tests of intelligence, development, attitudes, and vocational interests, and Buros's *The Eighth Mental Measurements Yearbook* (1978), which contains reviews of the tests and references regarding their use. Other sources for tests are the catalogs from the major test publishers. A list of bibliographic sources for tests is given in Appendix F.

Tests, measures, and inventories include those that are standardized and those that are non-standardized. Standardized tests are those that have been subjected to a process called

---

Box 7–H

For example, in a study measuring the range of motion in the affected elbow joint of patients with hemiplegia following a certain treatment technique, range of motion at the elbow could be operationally defined as the number of degrees registered on a goniometer placed on the joint angle while in extension and in flexion.

normalizing, which establishes a level of validity and reliability in relation to the "normal" population.

Validity

To say that a test is valid is to say that it measures what it claims to measure; for example, an intelligence test truly measures a child's intelligence rather than his or her school performance or his or her concentration and motivation.

Reliability

To say a test is reliable is to say that it will measure in the same manner and result in the same answers when measuring the same characteristic, time after time. For example, an intelligence test that is reliable will give the same intelligence quotient score for the same individual, time after time, all else being equal.

There are three types of reliability relevant to testing:

1. *Test-retest reliability* is concerned with the reliability of scores over time. Subjects are measured on some characteristic, a period of time is allowed to elapse, and the same subjects are remeasured on the same characteristic. The scores of the two administrations are then examined and, assuming that the conditions and the characteristic being measured are stable, the scores should be similar.
2. *Split-half reliability* concerns the extent to which different parts of an instrument are measuring the same thing. For instance, are two different items on a test for self-esteem both actually measuring components of self-esteem? If not, the whole test may be suspect, and the compiled score may not truly represent the subject's self-esteem score. To assess this type of reliability, the test is divided into two parts and subjects' scores on the two groups of items are compared. The two scores should be similar in order to consider the test reliable.
3. *Interrater reliability* is the extent to which different raters or observers perceive the same person or characteristic similarly. There are two parts to this concept: first, are observers consistent in their ratings within themselves, and second, are observers consistent in their ratings with other observers? Here again, ratings should be similar if observers are to be considered reliable.

The manual that accompanies a standardized test should include information about the process by which norms are established, details of the population used as normative groups, and the actual degree of validity and reliability established for the test. You should review this information to see if the test is rigorous enough for the purpose of your study. It is important that you use that test only on the type of subjects described in the manual. The researcher must learn the test administration procedures, and the test should be given only in the manner described in the manual. The reliability and validity of a test can be ensured only if the test is administered to the prescribed population, under the prescribed conditions, and in the prescribed manner. Once any of these items has been changed, the investigator cannot claim for his or her particular study the degree of reliability and validity listed in the manual.

DATA ANALYSIS

The data that have been gleaned may be qualitative or quantitative. Analysis of quantitative data will be taken up in Chapter 8, while analysis of qualitative data will be discussed here.

Qualitative data are usually generated from descriptive research. Case studies, ethnographies, historical and evaluation research usually generate large amounts of descriptive, non-quantifiable material that needs to be organized and synthesized in a useful manner. The data from interviews and questionnaires may be straightforward and simple to tabulate and analyze if they are generated from closed-ended questions, or may, if generated from open-ended questions, yield a mass of data in no particular format, which will be difficult to reduce to meaningful frequencies for analysis and interpretation.

CODING

Information received from open-ended questions can be subjected to a procedure called coding, which will make it easier to handle. First, a decision must be made whether to apply the *a priori* or *a posteriori* methods, which are described by Schwartzberg (1982). In the a posteriori approach "the categories of analysis are extracted from the material itself rather than being based upon a previously defined and outlined 'schematic system'" (p. 12). In the a priori approach "defined categories are decided upon beforehand, and then, data obtained is [sic] sorted by these categories" (p. 12).

Then the actual coding technique must be decided upon and may include word or concept coding:

1. Word coding is a technique in which the researcher selects key words that represent variables of interest to the researcher. The analysis consists of going through the data looking for the occurrence and frequency of the key words.
2. In concept coding, the researcher has a concept or idea in mind and notes each time that concept is mentioned by respondents. This process is more difficult than word coding because the concept can be elusive, and it takes great concentration to decide if specific groups of words comprise the concept. Concept coding requires training, expertise, patience, and perseverance.

CASE STUDY ANALYSIS

For case studies, there are three commonly used methods of analyzing data: Pattern matching, explanation building, and time-series analysis (Yin, 1989).

Pattern Matching

Using pattern-matching logic, an empirically based pattern (your findings) is compared with a predicted pattern (your hypothesis about the study variables). Predicted patterns may concern the dependent or the independent variables, either individually or with both interconnected. The researcher predicts a pattern of outcomes (a hypothesis), then matches the actual pattern of outcomes that has occurred. If the results are as predicted, you can draw a solid conclusion about the topic at hand, and you have substantiated your hypothesis. If the resulting pattern does not match the hypothesized pattern, you must re-evaluate your proposition (see Box 7-I).

Box 7-I

In a study concerning the use of electromechanical aids with severely retarded adults who have physical impairments (Bailey, 1990), it was hypothesized that such aids could be used to benefit this group (1) by enabling them to explore their environment, (2) by increasing their level of functioning, and (3) because previously these devices have been successfully used by other disabled clients. These hypothesized patterns were matched with the patterns found in the case study results of three women who had benefited from the use of electromechanical aids.

Explanation Building

Explanation building consists of analyzing data by building an explanation and stating a set of causal links about the case. This is usually preliminary to developing ideas and hypotheses for further study, and the explanations usually reflect some theoretically significant propositions. For example, public policy propositions can lead to recommendations for future policy actions. This is a difficult type of analysis to execute because the researcher is tempted to drift away from the original purpose of the study while explanations are being developed.

Explanation building is different from pattern matching in that, in the former, the explanation may not have been stated in the hypothesis at the beginning of the study. In a multicase study, the goal of explanation building is to build a general explanation that fits all cases (see Box 7–J).

Time-Series Analysis

Time-series analysis postulates a change or trend over time, and data are collected and analyzed at given points throughout the study, often annually. Then the original prediction is compared with the series of events actually recorded. This method is similar to pattern matching, but here the matching occurs over time rather than during one period at the end of the study (see Box 7–K).

The analysis of chronological events may be considered a special form of time-series analysis. This technique is a strength of case studies and allows analysis over a period of time. The analytic goal is to compare the actual chronology with that predicted by the researcher's theory. The theory will have specified one or more of the following kinds of conditions:

- Some events must always occur before other events (with the reverse being impossible)
- Some events must always be followed by other events on a contingency basis
- Some events can follow other events only after a prespecified passage of time, or
- Certain time periods in a case study may be marked by classes of events that differ substantially from those of other periods. (Yin, 1989)

If the sequence of events in the actual case study differ from the predicted sequence, the case can become the base for causal inferences; that is, new theory can be generated.

The important objective of the time-series approach to data analysis is to examine relevant "how" and "why" questions about the relationship of events over time, not merely to observe time trends alone. If a study is limited to a description of time trends, and no causal questions are asked or answered, then this is a non-case study. In other words, an essential feature of case studies is the generation of causal theory that can be tested using an experimental research design at a later date.

None of these case study data analysis strategies is easy to use, and none can be

---

Box 7–J

"In Derthick's *New towns in-town: Why a federal program failed* (1972), the federal government was to give its surplus land . . . to local governments for housing developments. But after four years, little progress had been made at the seven sites . . . and the program was considered a failure. Derthick's account first analyzes the events at each of the seven sites. Then, a general explanation—that the projects failed to generate sufficient support—is found unsatisfactory because the condition was not dominant at all of the sites. According to Derthick, although local support did exist, 'federal officials had nevertheless stated such ambitious objectives that some degree of failure was certain' (p. 91). Thus Derthick builds a modified explanation and concludes that 'the surplus lands program failed both because the federal government had limited influence at the local level and because it set impossibly high objectives'" (p. 93).

(Yin, 1989, p. 114)

Box 7 – K

To use Maude's case (presented in Box 5 – H) as an example, certain changes in Maude's abilities could have been predicted to happen at certain stages and in a specific chronology following the program of sensory training — changes (such as facial expression preceding speech) that were followed by orientation to place and person. It should be noted that this is not what the authors chose to do, but is used as an example of what could have occurred if a time-series analysis of the data had been used.

---

applied mechanically. Data analysis is the most difficult part of performing case studies and beginning investigators are especially likely to have a troublesome experience. It is recommended that the beginner start with a simple, straightforward case study before moving to more complicated cases.

ETHNOGRAPHY ANALYSIS

There are three popular methods for analyzing data obtained from ethnographical studies: triangulation, content analysis, and key event analysis.

Triangulation

Triangulation is a way of verifying validity, of testing one source of information against another in order to strip away alternative explanations and prove a hypothesis. Typically the ethnographer compares information sources to test the quality of the information (and the person sharing it) in order to put the whole situation into perspective.

Content Analysis

As described earlier, content analysis is a process of analyzing data by looking for repeated words, phrases, or concepts. It can be performed by hand but is lately more frequently performed on a computer because these types of data lend themselves to electronic manipulation. Data can be sorted, compared, contrasted, aggregated, and synthesized very speedily on a computer. The process can lead to the development of patterns or themes.

Ethnographers are interested in looking for patterns of thought and behavior. Patterns are a form of ethnographic reliability. The ethnographer begins with a mass of undifferentiated ideas and behavior, then collects pieces of information, comparing, contrasting, and sorting gross categories until a discernible thought or behavior pattern becomes identifiable. Next, observations must be compared with this poorly defined model until exceptions to the rule emerge and variations on a theme are detectable. After further sorting and sifting to make a match between categories, the theme or pattern finally emerges.

Key Events

Key events are other items a researcher can use to provide a focus in analyzing a culture or program. Some images are clear representations of social activity and provide a tremendous amount of embedded meaning. In many cases, the key event is a metaphor for a way of life or a specific social value. The case conference is a key event in a rehabilitation hospital, just as the morning meeting is a focal point on a psychiatric in-patient unit. Key events are extraordinarily useful for analysis, helping the researcher understand a social group as well as providing an explanation of the culture for others.

When triangulation has been performed, and patterns of behavior and key events are investigated so as to form a coherent picture, crystallization generally occurs. This is the moment when things fall into place and the ethnographer has an accurate and revealing picture of what is happening in the culture or program.

This chapter has presented several important strategies for analyzing qualitative data. The potential analytic difficulties can be reduced if you have a general strategy in mind for the analysis. Then, you are encouraged to "play with the data" in order to define the specific strategy that is most appropriate (e.g., pattern matching or coding). Skill and patience are required to execute most of these methods well. Qualitative data analysis is definitely a skill that improves with practice. The next chapter will present the analysis of quantitative data.

STUMBLING BLOCKS

A common problem in making observations is the inability to be impartial or objective, especially if the observer is also the main investigator, the one whose study is being observed. We all have the tendency to see what we want to see and this is often true of the researcher who wishes to see positive results in his or her research study. For this reason, it is a good idea to have more than one observer watching and recording the same event and, if possible, the person responsible for designing the study should not make the observations. It is also desirable for the observers to be ignorant of the hypothesis of the study, and to know as little as possible about the premises behind the study so that this information will not bias what they see. They also should not know whether subjects are in the experimental or control group while they are making observations. Observer bias is one of the major problems affecting the internal validity of a study, and the researcher should do everything possible to eliminate that bias. Oyster, Hanten, and Llorens (1987) offer an excellent segment on observer bias in *Introduction to Research: A Guide for the Health Science Professional.*

In designing a questionnaire, often the temptation is to adopt the attitude that "as long as I'm at it, why don't I ask . . ." and to add on a few more questions just because the questioner is curious. The temptation to ask for material that will not serve any useful purpose to the study should be overcome. Not only is it a waste of respondents' time, but it may serve to irritate them or cause them to run out of patience. A golden rule in survey construction is "Do not ask for information unless you can act on it" (Fink & Kosecoff, 1985, p. 25). This rule also applies to asking questions that will raise hopes you cannot fulfill (see Box 7–L).

Do not be too personal. A respondent may find the following questions insulting: "Are you divorced, married or single?" "How much money do you make in a year?" "How do you feel about your therapist?" If respondents find these questions too personal, either they will not answer them, or they will not answer them honestly. When personal information is essential to a survey, there are ways to phrase the questions to make them more tolerable, such as:

Box 7–L
"In a survey of a community's needs for health services, it would be unfair to have people rate their preference for a 24-hour emergency room staffed continuously by physicians if the community were unable to support such a service. Remember that the content of a survey can affect respondents' views and expectations." (Fink & Kosecoff, 1985, p. 25)

In which category was your salary last year?

(a) Below $10,000

(b) Between $10,000 and $20,000

(c) Between $20,000 and $30,000

(d) Between $30,000 and $40,000

(e) Over $40,000

Be careful not to lead respondents into giving you the answer they think you want. This may be done by adding positive or negative inferences to topics. For example, if you ask a subject about "working hard on a job," it implies that the job is hard when the subject may not view it that way.

While conducting a formal interview, the issue of pacing is important. There is the danger of moving too quickly because the interviewer is familiar with the material and does not need as much time as the subject to think about the questions. If the interview is rushed, subjects may feel unimportant, as if there is insufficient time for them. Subjects also need time to fully understand the questions and to think about their answers.

WORKSHEETS

Review the methods of data collection presented in this chapter and decide which methods you will be using:

_____ Observation

_____ Interview

_____ Questionnaire

_____ Record review

_____ Hardware

_____ Tests, measures, inventories

Remember that you may need to use more than one method to collect the necessary data for your study.

Observation: If you are using observation:
Which hypothesis do you plan to address with the observation?

What events, items, behaviors need to be observed?

Write an observable definition for each item.

What method will be used to record the observations? Sketch out a data collection chart/protocol.

Who will actually do the observing and recording?

Will they need training?

_____ Yes _____ No

If so, who will do the training?

Design a training procedure:

If there is more than one observer, will you test for interrater reliability?

_____ Yes _____ No

Describe the procedure you will use:

How will you tabulate the data from the observation? (Refer to the data collection protocol.)

What method will you use to analyze the data?

_____ Coding

_____ Pattern matching

_____ Explanation building

_____ Time-series analysis

_____ Triangulation

_____ Content analysis

_____ Key events

_____ Other

Interview or questionnaire: If you plan to use an interview or questionnaire to gather data:

Which hypothesis do you plan to address with the interview or questionnaire?

What specific information will you need in order to address this hypothesis?

What demographic data will you need in order to determine if the sample is representative of the population?

_____ Will you conduct the interview in person?

_____ Over the telephone?

_____ Will you use a written questionnaire to be left with subjects?

_____ Will you mail out a questionnaire?

_____ Will the interview be structured?

_____ Unstructured?

If you are mailing a questionnaire, compose the cover letter. Remember to include:

- Why the survey will be of interest and benefit to respondents
- The main goal for the survey
- A deadline for returning the questionnaire
- A stamped, self-addressed envelope

Make the cover letter and survey attractive.

You are now ready to compose the questions. First, decide on the exact pieces of data you need to know. Then, decide which format would best suit the question (e.g., yes/no format or multiple choice). Spend time on this until you feel you have the wording exactly right.

Conduct a small pilot study to see if your questions elicit the type of information you expected and if they are clear and unambiguous to respondents. (Read the section on pilot studies before doing this.)

Rewrite the questions based on the feedback from the pilot study.

How will you tabulate results?

_____ By hand

_____ By computer

What methods will you use to analyze data?

_____ Quantitative (see Chapter 8)

_____ Qualitative

If qualitative, list each question and define exactly which data analysis method will be used (e.g., coding, triangulation):

Record Review: If you plan to use a record review to gather data:

Which hypothesis will the record review address?

What data will you need to address this hypothesis?

Where will you find this information (specify for each):

Written material?

Physical material?

Mechanical material?

Which are primary sources?

Secondary sources?

Do you have sufficient primary sources to make this a viable method of data collection?

_____ Yes _____ No

What methods will you use to analyze the data?

_____ Coding

_____ Pattern matching

_____ Explanation building

_____ Triangulation

_____ Content analysis

_____ Other

Specify for each group of data which method you will use and how:

Hardware: If you plan to use hardware to gather data:

Which hypothesis will you address with the hardware?

What data do you need to gather in order to address this hypothesis?

Is there existing hardware to provide this data?

_____ Yes _____ No

Or will you have to develop your own?

_____ Yes _____ No

For existing hardware, is it standardized?

_____ Yes _____ No

_____ If so, what is the level of reliability?
_____ Validity?

If you are developing your own hardware, can you standardize it?

_____ Yes _____ No

If yes, describe the procedure:

What methods will you use to tabulate data?

What methods will you use to analyze data? (If quantitative, see next chapter.)

Tests, measures, inventories: If you plan to use tests, measures, or inventories to collect data:

Which hypothesis will be addressed by a test/measure/inventory?

What data do you need in order to address this hypothesis?

Is there an existing test that will elicit this data? _____ Yes _____ No

If yes, is it standardized? _____ Yes _____ No

_____ If yes, what is the level of reliability?
_____ Validity?

What is the scoring procedure?

Contact the publisher to find out if the test is available.

If you are constructing your own test, will you be able to standardize it?

_____ Yes _____ No

Construct the test, using the Benson and Clark (1982) article as a reference.

Conduct a pilot study and rework the test items based on the feedback. (Read section on pilot studies.)

What is the scoring procedure?

REFERENCES

Bailey, D. M. (1990). *Electromechanical aids in the treatment of multi-handicapped adults: A trilogy of case reports.* Unpublished paper.

Benson, J., & Clark, F. (1982). A guide for instrument development and validation. *American Journal of Occupational Therapy, 36*(12), 789–800.

Buros, O. K. (Ed.). (1975). *Tests in print II: An index to tests, test reviews, and the literature on specific tests.* Highland Park, NJ: Gryphon Press.

Buros, O. K. (Ed.). (1978). *The eighth mental measurements yearbook.* Highland Park, NJ: Gryphon Press.

Chun, K. T., Cobb, S., & French, J. R. (1985). *Measures for psychological assessment.* Ann Arbor, MI: Institute for Social Research, University of Michigan.

Converse, J. M., & Presser, S. (1986). *Survey questions: Handcrafting the standardized questionnaire.* No. 63 in Quantitative Applications in the Social Sciences Series. Newbury Park, CA: Sage Publications.

Currier, D. P. (1984). *Elements of research in physical therapy.* Baltimore: Williams & Wilkins.

Derthick, M. (1972). *New towns in-town: Why a federal program failed.* Washington, DC: Urban Institute.

Fink, A., & Kosecoff, J. (1985). *How to conduct surveys: A step-by-step guide.* Beverly Hills, CA: Sage Publications.

Hemphill, B. J. (1982). *The evaluative process in psychiatric occupational therapy.* Thorofare, NJ: Slack.

Henry, A. D., Nelson, D. L., & Duncombe, L. W. (1984). Choice making in group and individual activity. *American Journal of Occupational Therapy, 38*(4), 245–251.

Likert, R. (1932). A technique for the measurement of attitudes. *Archives of Psychology, 52,* 140–145.

Osgood, C., Suci, G., & Tannenbaum, P. (1957). *The measurement of meaning.* Urbana, IL: University of Illinois Press.

Oyster, C., Hanten, W., & Llorens, L. (1987). *Introduction to research: A guide for the health science professional.* Philadelphia: J.B. Lippincott.

Robinson, J. P., & Shriver, P. R. (1985). *Measures of social psychological attitudes.* Ann Arbor, MI: Institute for Social Research, University of Michigan.

Schuman, H., & Presser, S. (1981). *Questions and answers in attitude surveys: Experiments on question form, wording, and context.* New York: Academic Press.

Schwartzberg, S. (1982). Motivation for activities of daily living: A study of selected psychiatric patients' self-reports. *Occupational Therapy in Mental Health, 2*(3), 1–26.

Stein, F. (1989). *Anatomy of clinical research: An introduction to scientific inquiry in medicine, rehabilitation and related health professions.* Thorofare, NJ: Slack, Inc.

Yin, R. K. (1989). *Case study research: Design and methods.* No. 5 in Applied Social Science Research Methods Series. Newbury Park, CA: Sage Publications.

ADDITIONAL READING

Converse, J. M., & Presser, S. (1986). *Survey questions: Handcrafting the standardized questionnaire.* No. 63 in Quantitative Applications in the Social Sciences Series. Newbury Park, CA: Sage Publications.

Ethridge, D., & McSweeney, M. (1971). Research in occupational therapy: 4. Data collection and analysis. *American Journal of Occupational Therapy, XXV*(2), 90–97.

Fink, A., & Kosecoff, J. (1985). *How to conduct surveys: A step-by-step guide.* Beverly Hills, CA: Sage Publications.

Schuman, H., & Presser, S. (1981). *Questions and answers in attitude surveys: Experiments on question form, wording, and context.* New York: Academic Press.

Weber, R. (1985). *Basic content analysis.* No. 49 in Quantitative Applications in the Social Sciences Series. Newbury Park, CA: Sage Publications.

Analyzing Quantitative Data

Next is the part that many people hate! What to do with this mass of numbers that have been collected? What statistical manipulations to apply? Some people have such a fear of this part of the research process that they never get beyond it. The fear and/or lack of knowledge may be real or imagined but should not be allowed to stand in the way of the therapist as a researcher. If you feel at all uncertain about quantitative data analysis, you are advised to get help from a statistician.

CONSULTING A STATISTICIAN

Consulting a statistician will have a price, but most people I know who have hired someone feel it is worth the cost. You may be fortunate enough to be connected to a university or a facility that employs a statistician who is willing to help free of charge or for a nominal fee. Otherwise, you may have to contact a statistician (call your local college or university for suggestions) and inquire about charges; hourly rates may be quite high, so it will pay to shop around.

The question of when to seek statistical assistance during the research process is worthy of discussion. A statistician should be consulted in the design stage of the project, while you are still deciding on the instruments or measures you will use to collect data. You will be the one to decide on the actual measures used and whether these measures will collect the type of data you want as reliably as you wish. However, the statistician understands how the data will be analyzed and may have some advice concerning the format in which the data is to be collected.

For example, in knowing that you wish to compare two groups' performances on pre-tests and post-tests in order to determine which group made the most progress, the statistician may advise that data resulting from a certain measure are not in a format suitable for such comparisons. An unclear response from subjects such as, "I feel somewhat better," does not lend itself to objective comparisons, either for that one subject or among subjects.

More often, some crucial piece of information concerning subjects has been omitted from a questionnaire—for instance, their ages. If you wish to group people in age groups for comparisons, this information will be important. Although the therapist obviously has the ability to spot this type of error, it sometimes takes an objective reader who is accustomed to studying data to notice it.

Assisting the therapist in designing formats for the collection of data is another way the statistician can be helpful. Knowing how the data will be entered on a computer, for instance, allows the statistician to understand that this will be more easily accomplished if numbers are arranged linearly with a separate line for each subject.

Finally, a statistician may see that a certain statistical test will be best suited to achieve the analysis you wish to make, and can advise on how many subjects are needed in order to use that test. You would want this information early in the planning stages of your project. Thus, it can be seen that seeking assistance from a statistician early on in the research design process is helpful in ensuring that data will be collected in such a way that they can be manipulated effectively.

Anything but basic statistics is beyond the scope of this manual. However, it is hoped that a simple explanation of some of the processes involved in organizing and manipulating data will enable the reader with "statistics fear" to cope with the material—and to know when to get help.

DESCRIPTIVE VERSUS INFERENTIAL STATISTICS

Statistics may conveniently be divided into two categories: descriptive and inferential statistics. Descriptive statistics are those that describe, organize, and summarize data. They include such things as frequencies, percentages, descriptions of central tendency (mean, median, mode), and descriptions of relative position (range, standard deviation).

These procedures allow for the description of all the individual scores in a sample on one variable by using one or two numbers, such as the mean and the standard deviation. They can be used to describe each dependent variable, such as the percentage and mean of each item physical therapists checked off on a list of reasons for moving into supervisory positions and their ages when they moved. Descriptive statistics can also be used to give the variation or spread of scores within each group studied, such as the mean and range of scores for experimental and control groups in a study on a new treatment technique for carpal tunnel syndrome.

Inferential statistics, on the other hand, allow one to make inferences from the sample to the population in order to speculate, reason, and generalize about the population from the sample findings. Sufficient subjects are needed in the sample to be able to do this; in addition, random selection should be used. The types of statistical tests used in inferential statistics include t tests, F tests, and tests for r. These tests result in probability statements that help one draw conclusions about differences or relationships between groups. For example, if a difference is found between the mean scores of two groups at the end of a study, the researcher must decide whether a similar difference is likely to be found between the same mean scores in the whole population—the t, F, and r tests would allow the researcher to make this decision.

Both descriptive and inferential statistics are often used in the same research study. Descriptive statistical methods are the same whether parametric or non-parametric data are being used; however, inferential statistical methods will vary according to the type of data used. For this statement to be understood, the terms *parametric* and *non-parametric* need to be explained.

PARAMETRIC AND NON-PARAMETRIC DATA

The data that have been collected in your study may be characterized in four different ways: nominal, ordinal, interval, and ratio.

NOMINAL DATA

Nominal data are the numbers applied to non-numerical variables (e.g., eye color may be coded as follows: blue = 1, brown = 2, hazel = 3, etc.). Each category of data must be mutually exclusive, meaning that no individual or variable could be assigned to more than one group. There is no ordered relationship between categories, meaning that one category could not be considered to come before or after another category. This type of data is sometimes referred to as "discrete" as opposed to "continuous." There is no limit to the number of categories that can be included in a nominal scale. Because there is no numerical value to categories, they cannot be meaningfully added, subtracted, or multiplied, and so forth. One cannot calculate an average (mean) eye color, for example.

Examples of categories are: male and female; goniometers and dynomometers; patients with schizophrenia, bipolar disease, or depression; patients with right hemiplegia or left hemiplegia. A nominal scale may also be used to code such responses on a survey as "yes/no" or "never/sometimes/always."

ORDINAL DATA

Ordinal data are numbers that still are discrete but are ordered. However, the intervals between the categories are not known and cannot be assumed to be equal. Numbers can be assigned to groups, and the numbers can be put into a meaningful sequence. For instance, a review committee may rank-order a series of program proposals and assign first, second, and third place, but the top-ranked proposal may be considerably better than the ones ranked second and third, while the ones ranked fourth, fifth, and sixth may be similar to each other in quality. These differences between intervals would not be reflected in the numerical assignment. Other examples would be ratings on a Likert scale such as Strongly agree, Agree, Neutral, Disagree, Strongly disagree; or classifications for client ability such as Needs full assist, Partial assist, Independent. An ordinal data scale indicates a greater or lesser degree of something, or it may reflect a "precedes" or "superior" concept.

INTERVAL DATA

Interval data also are ordered in a logical sequence. However, this time the intervals between the numbers are considered equal and represent actual amounts. These are continuous data. Examples are intelligence scores, degrees of muscle strength, and degrees of perceptual motor skills. Items are ordered on a continuum; however, there is no actual zero point. For instance, the zero reading on a dynamometer does not reflect a total absence of muscle strength — it is not a measure of anything.

RATIO DATA

Ratio data are numbers that also are continuous with equal intervals between numbers. Additionally, ratio data have a meaningful zero point. In other words, the zero point indicates a total absence of whatever ability or property is being measured. For instance, there legitimately can be zero range of motion or visual acuity. "Ratio data can be multiplied and divided, enabling one to say that a range of motion of 40 degrees is twice that of a 20-degree range" (Hasselkus & Safrit, 1976, p. 431).

Nominal and ordinal data are known as non-parametric data, while interval and ratio data are parametric data. The importance of making this distinction is that one will know what kind of statistics can be used to manipulate these data. While most of the descriptive statistics can be used on both parametric and non-parametric data (the exception being that means and standard deviations cannot be used on nominal data), different inferential statistics must be used on the two types of data. This is due to the properties of the data, such as being ordered, or such as the intervals between numbers being equal. Some tests are not powerful enough to cope with unordered, unequal data, while others are. Nominal data need such non-parametric tests as the chi-square or Mann-Whitney tests, while interval data can be manipulated using *t* tests and analyses of variance. Table 8–1 may be helpful in

Table 8–1.
Categories of Data with Corresponding Classifications and Inferential Tests

Categories of Data	Classification	Examples of Inferential Tests
Nominal data: named categories, unordered	Non-parametric	Pearson's chi-square Fisher's exact Goodman and Kruskal's tau b
Ordinal data: ordered categories, unequal intervals	Non-parametric	Pearson's chi-square Spearman rho Wilcoxon rank sum Mann-Whitney Kruskal-Wallis Kendall's tau
Interval data: ordered data with equal intervals between categories	Parametric	t tests Analysis of variance (ANOVA) Analysis of covariance (ANCOVA)
Ratio data: equal intervals with zero point	Parametric	t tests Analysis of variance (ANOVA) Pearson product moment correlation

summarizing categories of data with their corresponding classifications and types of statistical tests.

There are some rules that need to be applied to the distribution of data in order to be able to use parametric tests:

1. The sample must be representative of the target population so that the variables being measured fall within the normal distribution for that population (for example, random selection has occurred).
2. Variables must have been measured in a manner that generates interval or ratio data.
3. Initial differences between subjects in the two groups under study must have the opportunity to be similar (i.e., random assignment to groups or matching must have occurred).

When any of these conditions has not been met, non-parametric statistics should be used; that is, when:

1. Random selection has not occurred, so that the sample is not considered representative of the population and variables are probably not normally distributed.
2. Variables have been measured in a manner that generates nominal or ordinal data.
3. The numbers of subjects in the sample are small.

Because non-parametric data do not meet strict statistical criteria, substantial differences must be found between sets of scores before those differences are considered meaningful.

It is frequently the case that non-parametric statistics should be used in health science research, because pathological human conditions are being studied. The variables of illness or pathology often are not distributed normally in the target population. Also, it is often difficult to locate many subjects with the requisite pathology, so sample groups tend to be small.

DESCRIPTIVE STATISTICS

A great deal of quantitative data can be effectively analyzed using descriptive statistics. In fact, if a non-experimental research design is employed, almost all of the data will be appropriately analyzed descriptively because random selection may not have been used for the sample and there may not be a control group. It is difficult to make inferences from a sample to a population (the purpose of inferential statistics) if random sampling and control criteria have not been met.

The initial description and compilation of data can be achieved using descriptive statistics, that is, providing the frequencies, percentages, and means for all the characteristics under study so that the reader has a thorough understanding of the subjects and variables. It is customary to present percentages alongside the frequencies, both in the text and in illustrative tables.

It is often useful to give the reader the group's average score, that is, their *central tendency*. The mean, median, or mode can be used to describe central tendency. The mean is computed by adding all the scores and dividing the total by the number in the group. The median is the midpoint between all the scores. Each score must be listed before finding the midpoint, which incidentally may end up not being a whole number. The mode is the most commonly occurring score. There may be more than one mode; for instance, in a list of IQ scores, four people may score 110 and four people may score 115. In this instance, the total group of scores would be referred to as bimodal. Oyster, Hanten, and Llorens (1987) provide a useful description of when to use which of the measures of central tendency.

The reader also may wish to know the *relative position* of subjects and their scores. For instance, a range will explain the section of the continuum in which the subjects scored, perhaps IQ scores from 90 to 120, resulting in a range of 31. Another way to describe relative position is to use the standard deviation, referred to as s or SD. The standard deviation indicates how the scores are grouped around the midpoint. To continue using the IQ example, a group of 7-year-olds with a mean IQ of 100 whose scores ranged from 90 to 110 would be quite different from a group of 7-year-olds with a mean IQ of 100 whose scores ranged from 70 to 120.

There are many useful ways to illustrate descriptive data, such as tables, pie charts, and graphs. These formats are described in Chapter 10.

INFERENTIAL STATISTICS

Inferential statistics are those that allow us to take the results from a research project and decide whether those findings are likely to occur in the target population. Inferential statistics are used to help us decide the chances of that occurring. If there is a statistically significant result, we may decide that the probability is great that we have in fact found a result that can be generalized to the target population.

Tests for inferential statistics can be divided into three groups:

1. Those that try to find if the differences observed between two sets of scores are significantly different
2. Those that examine two sets of scores to find the strength of association between them
3. Those tests that compare more than two sets of scores to find the extent to which they vary together.

SIGNIFICANT DIFFERENCES

In this group, the tests assist the researcher in deciding whether the changes in the mean scores of the experimental group are, in fact, due to the experimental treatment, rather than due to chance. They allow comparison of results from the sample with that which was hypothesized as normally occurring in the target population. The tests can be used with a directional hypothesis or with a two-sided hypothesis.

To use the classic experimental research design as an example:

$$R \quad O_1 \quad X \quad O_2$$
$$R \quad O_3 \quad \quad O_4$$

statistical difference tests would be applied to the scores from the pre- and post-test results of the experimental results (O_1 and O_2), and to the pre- and post-test scores of the control

---

Box 8–A

An example of the classic experimental design can be found in Mitchell, Daines, and Thomas's (1987) study of the effects of ingestion of amino acids on burning pain threshold. One experimental group received L-tryptophan, a second experimental group received Phenylalanine, and a control group received a placebo. At pre-testing, the three groups showed a wide difference in "normal" pain threshold, so a statistical test was used at the end of the study (analysis of covariance, ANCOVA), which could adjust the post-test scores, based on those differences. In measuring the results of the three groups on the post-test, the ANCOVA showed that there was no significant difference between the groups.

---

group (O_3 and O_4), and finally to the post-test scores of the two groups (O_2 and O_4). The first result would indicate the degree of change following the experimental treatment, the second would indicate changes following no treatment, and the third result would show the difference between end conditions of the experimental and control groups. If the difference between the scores on the third test (between O_2 and O_4) were statistically significant, it would indicate that changes could be attributed to the treatment rather than to chance (see Box 8–A).

Significance testing is based on the laws of probability. It answers the question: What is the probability that this change occurred because of events in the research study, and what is the probability that this change would have occurred anyway, by chance? The tests that are used to make this determination result in a level of probability, and it is the researcher who decides whether or not this level is significant. In the social sciences, the usual convention is that 5 occurrences in 100 of the change being due to chance is a reasonable number to accept, and that any result better than that is statistically significant. This result would imply that it is 95 percent certain that the improvement in post-test scores was caused by the treatment. This probability level is expressed as $p < .05$. Some scientific endeavors require more stringent proof, and a standard of $p < .01$, or one chance in a hundred that the change occurred by chance, is set for those studies, otherwise seen as a 99 percent success rate. Clinicians must decide on the significance level to be used, deciding how acceptable it would be for the dependent variable to be changed by the independent variable at various levels of certainty (see Box 8–B).

The tests most commonly used to determine significance levels are Pearson's chi-square test on non-parametric (nominal and ordinal) data and the student's t test on parametric (interval and ratio) data. The chi-square and t tests can be used to compare two groups on only one variable at a time.

Pearson's Chi-Square Test

In the Pearson's chi-square test, the data used for analysis are counts of category membership (e.g., How many subjects are men and how many are women? or How many have blue

---

Box 8–B

A decision concerning significance level was made by physical therapists when they were studying the relationship between infant neuromotor assessment and preschool motor measures. In the research design section of their article, the authors state:

> Because we used multiple comparisons, the alpha level was set at .01. This level also was thought to be advisable because, with a sample size of 77, correlation coefficients could be large enough to be significant at the .05 level but not large enough to be clinically significant. (Deitz, Crowe, & Harris, 1987, p. 15)

Here, the clinicians are making a decision about the level of significance based on the idiosyncrasies of a specific test (Spearman's rank correlation coefficients).

Box 8-C

Coren and colleagues (1987) investigated the factors related to physical therapy students' decisions to work with elderly patients. They used chi-square tests to determine relationships between students' intentions to work with the elderly and their answers to questions concerned with such things as biographical information (students' age, whether they had ever lived with their grandparents, whether they had friends over the age of 65 years), experiential influences (courses in problems of the elderly, weekly home visits with the well elderly, clinical rotations in a geriatric setting), and attitudinal perceptions (concern that salaries might be lower in geriatric settings, lack of prestige in working with the elderly). Answers to the questions were of the nominal and ordinal type, so that chi-square tests were appropriate for data analyses.

---

eyes and how many have brown eyes?) Pearson's chi-square test may be used when you wish to know if there are significant differences between pre-test and post-test scores for a given group, or if you wish to know if two groups are similar when you intend to use one as an experimental group and one as a control group. It can be used to compare groups on a single variable or on groups of variables, one at a time. This test is useful when the researcher is interested in similarities between groups of subjects (see Box 8-C). If the researcher can determine the numbers of characteristics such as gender, age, or eye color, a chi-square test on the respondents will test whether the sample matches the population. The calculated value for the chi-square formula is evaluated using standardized tables that list critical values. When the chi-square exceeds the table value, the hypothesis is supported.

t Tests

There are three different t tests, each of which is used with a different research design, but all compare the mean scores of two groups. The single sample t test compares the mean for a sample against a known population mean for a particular variable. This test is rarely used because the mean score for a population is rarely available. The paired groups t test is used when subjects have been used as their own control group and when groups consist of individuals who have been matched on some characteristic. In this case, the pre-test and post-test scores are compared for the first group and the two scores from the matched pairs are compared for the second group. In the independent groups t test, the pre-test and post-test means are compared for the experimental and control groups, and the two post-test scores are compared. This is the most commonly used t test (see Box 8-D).

If you have decided on a direction for your hypothesis, a one-tailed t test should be used to determine significance of results. If a non-directional hypothesis has been used, a two-tailed t test should be employed to determine the direction of the significance, if any (see Box 8-E). The t test is quite powerful and can be used on groups of subjects smaller than 30.

Wilcoxon Signed Rank Test

The Wilcoxon signed rank test is used on non-parametric data and is equivalent to the correlated groups t test. It is performed on paired scores and will determine the significance of the difference between either pre-test and post-test scores for individuals (see Box 8-F) or scores on matched pairs of subjects.

Box 8-D

Shinabarger (1987) used an independent group t test to compare the range of motion scores for each of eight motions between subjects with diabetes mellitus in experimental and control groups.

Box 8–E

Liu, Currier, and Threlkeld (1987) investigated the effects of electrical stimulation on the blood circulation of an unexercised part of the body. They used an independent, two-tailed t test to determine equality between the experimental and control groups, to analyze the pre-stimulated heart rate, blood pressure, and pulsatility index. They found that the groups were similar on these variables before experimental intervention and thus did not need to make adjustments later via statistical analyses.

Box 8–F

The Wilcoxon signed rank test was used in a study of the effects of a maternal preparation program on mother-infant pairs (Hamilton-Dodd, Kawamoto, Clark, Burke, & Fanchiang, 1989). Tests were performed separately on the experimental and control groups' prenatal and postnatal questionnaire scores.

Wilcoxon Rank Sum Test

The Wilcoxon rank sum test is the equivalent to the t test for independent groups, but is used on non-parametric data. For this test, ranks are assigned to scores for all subjects in the study, and the ranks for all subjects in each group are summed. The test will determine the degree of differences between group total scores (see Box 8–G).

Mann-Whitney Test

The Mann-Whitney test is yet a third alternative to the t test for use on non-parametric data. It tests for differences between means on two independent groups and is equivalent to the independent groups t test (see Box 8–H).

Box 8–G

Case-Smith, Cooper, and Scala (1989) used the Wilcoxon rank sum test "to estimate whether or not the differences between the summed scores were significant" (p. 247). The researchers compared efficient and non-efficient neonate feeders on neonatal oral motor assessment scores.

Box 8–H

In studying changes in students' perceptions of the professional role, Corb and colleagues (1987) employed a Mann-Whitney U test to investigate differences between students' and faculty members' perceptions of various concepts. Concepts related to professional role were investigated using a semantic differential technique with a seven-point scale, so that data generated were of the ordinal type (i.e., numerical values 1 through 7 representing respondents' agreement with one or other of the adjectives).

TESTS FOR CORRELATION

These tests are used to examine two sets of scores to find the extent of their relationship to one another. The two sets of scores might be from one set of individuals or from two different groups of individuals. Once it is seen that one score moves up or down, the intent is to find out if the other score moves in a corresponding fashion. The objective is to find out how closely the scores covary, that is, whether they change together in a particular pattern—in a positive or negative way. If both scores increase together, they are said to be positively correlated; for example, height and weight scores for a group of subjects would probably increase together. If, on the other hand, scores for age over 60 years and scores for muscle strength were computed, age scores might increase while strength scores decreased. These scores would be said to be negatively correlated. The two sets of scores that are being compared in correlation testing can be entered on a scattergram to show the degree of correlation graphically (see Box 8–I).

Tests for correlation yield a statistic called a correlation coefficient, expressed as r. An r may range from -1 (indicating a perfect negative relationship) to $+1$ (indicating a perfect positive relationship). A zero would indicate that there is no relationship between the two variables. Decimal factors are used to indicate r scores (i.e., .87 or $-.66$). As with the previous tests, a level of significance can be computed for an r score.

Pearson Product Moment Correlation

The most common correlation test is the Pearson product moment method, often called the Pearson r, which is used on parametric data. This test can be used on group scores or individual scores. It will indicate only systematic disagreements between scores and will not show the odd or occasional disagreement. It is often used to estimate reliability between tests, as in a test-retest situation, or between two testers to indicate intertester reliability (see Box 8–J).

Spearman Rho

The Spearman rho method is the equivalent to the Pearson r. It is used in descriptive research resulting in non-parametric data when items have been ranked and the investigator wishes to compare two sets of rankings to see if there is any type of relationship between them. Like the Pearson, it results in an r value falling between -1 and $+1$ (see Box 8–K).

It is important to remember that a relationship between two sets of scores does not necessarily mean that this is a cause-and-effect relationship. The researcher can claim only that a positive or negative relationship between the variables has been found, and no more.

Regression Analysis

Regression analysis is a technique that can be used after the correlation coefficient has been established. When a relationship has been found between two variables, one can

---

Box 8–I

Taylor and colleagues (1987) use the scattergram to good effect as discussed in their article on the effects of interferential current stimulation for treatment of subjects with recurrent jaw pain. The scattergram illustrates the intensity of mean jaw pain on the vertical axis and the subject groups on the horizontal axis.

Box 8–J

Gogia and colleagues (1987) investigated the intertester reliability of goniometric measurements at the knee and the validity of the clinical measurements by comparing the measurements taken from roentgenograms. They used the Pearson product-moment correlation coefficient to compare the measurements recorded by two therapists and to compare measurements obtained by each therapist to those derived from the roentgenograms.

Box 8–K

The authors of a study on the relationship between infant neuromotor assessment and preschool motor measures state clearly why they used the Spearman test:

> Because the assumptions for the use of parametric statistics were not met, the relationships were examined using Spearman's rank correlation coefficients. (p. 15)

(Deitz, Crowe, & Harris, 1987)

---

attempt to predict future scores for the dependent variable based on the scores on which the correlation coefficient was found.

COMPARISON OF MORE THAN TWO VARIABLES

As was mentioned in the section on factorial research, the investigator often wishes to explore more than two variables in the same study. In this case, different statistical tests are needed.

Analysis of Variance

Analysis of variance (ANOVA) is a statistical technique that can compare the mean scores of three or more groups in one study. It deals with multigroup questions, such as the one in Box 8–L.

The ANOVA yields an F ratio, which is evaluated using a standardized table to see if there is a significant difference between the largest and smallest of the study group means. If you wish to see if there are significant differences between any of the other means, you must use another test, such as the Duncan range test, the Newman-Keuls test, or the Tukey test (see Box 8–M).

In addition to informing the investigator of differences between the means of the study groups (e.g., differences between total means for the 5-, 6-, 7-, 8-, and 9-year-olds), the ANOVA can give information about differences between the individuals within each group. If each of the 5-year-olds, for instance, had 10 trials on each of the activities, a mean could be computed for each child and those means entered into the ANOVA equation. The test

---

Box 8–L

Is there a difference in bilateral motor coordination measured by jumping jacks, symmetrical stride jumps and reciprocal stride jumps, in 5- to 9-year-old children? (Magalhaes, Koomar, & Cermak, 1989). In this study there were five groups: 5-, 6-, 7-, 8-, and 9-year-olds, each divided into girls and boys. Each group of children was tested on the three activities (independent variables) to measure their abilities against existing tests for bilateral motor coordination. ANOVA was used to determine the effect of age and sex on the three activities. The tests were also capable of determining the interaction between age, sex, and task.

Box 8-M

Lohmann and colleagues (1987) found through an ANOVA that there were significant differences between mean measurements of tibia vara between limbs when the lower extremity was in different positions under different conditions and used a Newman-Keuls test to see exactly where the differences were — between which of the three groups.

---

would then compute whether there were significant differences among the 5-year-olds. ANOVA is powerful enough to be able to pick out odd or occasional differences in an individual's scores.

Analysis of Covariance

A similar test is the analysis of covariance (ANCOVA). It controls for initial differences between groups. If pre-test scores show that the dependent variable is substantially different for the groups due to extraneous variables such as age or sex, an ANCOVA can take into account the extraneous variables by treating them as covariates and by extracting their effect from the data. By making the groups more equitable to begin with, the final results can be compared and judged more fairly (see Box 8-N).

Kruskal-Wallis Test

The Kruskal-Wallis test is an equivalent test to the one-way ANOVA and can be used on non-parametric data. Like other non-parametric tests, this test is based on rankings of scores on the dependent measure in which all subjects are put into one group during the ranking procedure, then put back into their original treatment groups for the remaining analysis (see Box 8-O).

Multiple Regression

This test provides a way of making predictions about the study variable by understanding the effects of two or more independent variables on the study variable (i.e., How much do the independent variables correlate with the study variable?). It is possible to take the

---

Box 8-N

While testing for the possible effect of amino acids on burning pain threshold in two experimental groups and one control group, investigators used an ANCOVA to control statistically for the wide individual variance found in pre-test pain measures.
(Mitchell, Daines, & Thomas, 1987)

Box 8-O

When investigating the differences in perceptions among three groups of respondents who assessed the importance of 80 competencies for physical therapists treating patients with arthritis, Moncur (1987) used the Kruskal-Wallis one-way analysis of variance (ANOVA) to make group comparisons. Levels of importance of a competency were compared among the different practitioner groups by the Kruskal-Wallis ANOVA test.

procedure a step further by untangling the relative contributions of each of the independent variables. One can then use step-wise regression to look at the independent variables in various combinations to see which combination is most useful in predicting the occurrence of the study variable.

Only some of the many possible tests for manipulating data are reviewed here. A statistician will be familiar with other possibilities and will be able to advise on the appropriate statistical tests based on your specific research design.

COMPUTER ANALYSIS

All of the above tests can be computed by hand, but this is a tedious and time-consuming process and most people now use a computer for statistical processing. With the help of a statistician or a computer assistant, most therapists can enter the raw data onto the computer disk. It is also possible for therapists and students to perform the statistical manipulations by learning the entry keys for the relevant statistical software package. There are manuals for each package, but they are often difficult to follow without some basic computer literacy. Three commonly used statistical software packages designed for the health and social sciences are:

> SAS/STAT—SAS/STAT User's Guide, Version 6, ed. 4. SAS Institute, Inc., Cary, NC. (1989).
>
> SPSS—Statistical Package for the Social Sciences, M. J. Norusis, McGraw-Hill, New York. (1989).
>
> BMDP—Biomedical Data Package, University of California, Berkeley, CA. (1981).

A fourth package, Minitab, is an effective statistical analysis software package that was developed for use in introductory statistics courses. It has recently been made available for use on personal computers as The Student Edition of Minitab (Schaefer & Anderson, 1989). This edition comes with a clearly written manual and is powerful enough to do most of the statistical procedures likely to be used in therapists' and students' research studies. The program is summarized in the user's manual as follows: "An interactive statistical software package for organizing, analyzing, and reporting statistical data. Statistical features include basic statistics, regression analysis, analysis of variance, and nonparametric tests, among others, with graphics to enhance the display of data" (p. iv).

If you need to analyze more than just a small amount of data, using a computer is highly recommended. It is well worth the researcher's time to take a basic computer course to learn to move around the keyboard, to understand basic computer concepts, and to enter data.

All the work accomplished by the reader up to this point has been the planning for the actual research study. In the next chapter, we will look at some finishing touches and finally discuss carrying out the project itself.

STUMBLING BLOCKS

It is not easy to find a statistician with whom one is compatible and with whom one can communicate easily, but it is definitely worth the search and the cost. If you are not sure where to go for help, ask colleagues who have participated in research, or faculty at the local therapy training program. There is usually someone on the faculty whose job it is to assist with statistics, and he or she may be willing to work with private clients. Alternatively, you might be fortunate enough to find a fellow therapist or a colleague knowledgeable about statistics who can help you. Too often I have seen therapists or students struggling to understand a statistician and feeling that the problem was all their own. They

---

Box 8–P

"In a study of the efficacy of chest physiotherapy and intermittent positive pressure breathing in the resolution of pneumonia by Graham and Bradley (1978), the conclusion was that chest physiotherapy and intermittent positive pressure breathing do not hasten resolution of pneumonia. However, most therapists would not consider physiotherapy had a place in the treatment of acute pneumonia. The lack of statistically significant differences between treated and untreated groups was not of real life "significance" or importance."
(Partridge & Barnitt, 1986, p. 77)

Box 8–Q

"For example, in the pain study significantly more subjects might have preferred to read *Time* magazine than *Newsweek*. Although such a difference may be meaningful to the sales managers of these publications, this information probably has little relevance to the outcome of the pain experiment."
(Cohen, 1988, p. 599)

---

have been reluctant to ask questions or to change consultants. Of course, the problem is never one-sided. Often it is the statistician who does not understand the clinical process and who is unable to design data collection and analysis methods that are appropriate. Either way, it is best to leave that situation and find someone else. You may even have to try two or three people before finding the one who is right for you.

Be sure that you are clear in your own mind what it is you hope to find out as a result of the data analysis. For example, know if you want to determine the difference between pre-test and post-test results for the same group of subjects, or if you want to know the difference between two post-test results for two different groups of subjects. Sometimes therapists get talked into performing complex and elegant statistical manipulations on their data by statisticians who are more interested in proving that they can do such manipulations than they are in helping therapists achieve their goals. The analyses may look impressive but often do not make much sense in real-life terms in relation to the data. As Partridge and Barnitt (1986) state, "It is. . . important to distinguish 'real life' significance from 'statistical' significance—they may be different. . ." (p. 76). A useful example to illustrate the point is given as shown in Box 8–P. Cohen (1988) offers a further example of the concepts "significant" and "meaningful" not being synonymous, as presented in Box 8–Q.

Finally, I recommend again that you consult with a statistician before you begin to collect data, to ensure that all the necessary data are collected and that they are collected in a format that is useful.

WORKSHEETS

Review the research design and data collection methods you have selected for your project.

Are you using:
_____ An experimental design?

_____ A quasi-experimental design?

_____ A non-experimental design?

Are you collecting data using:
_____ Observation?

_____ Interview?

_____ Questionnaire?

_____ Record review?

_____ Equipment?

_____ Tests, measures, inventories?

Will you be confined to descriptive statistics or will you also be able to use inferential statistics?
_____ Descriptive?

_____ Inferential?

For the descriptive statistics, which ones do you think would help the reader to understand your results?
_____ Frequencies and percentages?

_____ Central tendency: mean, median, mode?

_____ Relative position: range, standard deviation?

For inferential statistics:

Will the results of the data collection techniques yield:
_____ Nominal data?

_____ Ordinal data?

_____ Interval data?

_____ Ratio data?

Therefore, will you be using parametric or non-parametric statistics to analyze your data?
_____ Parametric?

_____ Non-parametric?

Do you wish to test for:
_____ Significant differences between groups?

_____ Correlation between variables?

_____ A comparison of more than two variables?

What test(s) does it seem likely that you could use to make these determinations?
_____ t test(s)

_____ chi-square

_____ Wilcoxon signed rank test

_____ Wilcoxon rank sum test

_____ Mann-Whitney test

_____ Pearson product moment correlation

_____ Spearman rho

_____ Regression analysis

_____ ANOVA

_____ ANCOVA

_____ Kruskal-Wallis test

INFORMATION SHEET TO TAKE TO THE STATISTICIAN

In order to help the statistician understand what you wish to achieve in your study, take some basic information with you when you meet. The following information would give the statistician a clear idea of your project:

Hypotheses:

Subjects:

- How many?

- How selected?

- In how many groups?

- How assigned to groups?

Methods: Type of research design (e.g., pre-test/treatment/post-test; survey; comparison of experimental and control groups).

Specific data collection methods (e.g., self-designed questionnaire; IQ test; values inventory, goniometer readings).

Type of data that will be generated (nominal, ordinal, interval, ratio; more than one type). Give actual examples of data.

Your initial thoughts on data analysis:

If using descriptive statistics:

_____ Frequencies and percentages

_____ Central tendency

_____ Relative position

If using inferential statistics:

_____ Significance between groups

_____ Correlation between groups

_____ Comparison of more than one variable

Therefore, some thoughts on specific tests _____

_____

_____

REFERENCES

Case-Smith, J., Cooper, P., & Scala, V. (1989). Feeding efficiency of premature neonates. *American Journal of Occupational Therapy, 43*(4), 245–250.

Cohen, H. (1988). How to read a research paper. *American Journal of Occupational Therapy, 42*(9), 596–600.

Corb, D. F., Pinkston, D., Harden, R. S., O'Sullivan, P., & Fecteau, L. (1987). Changes in students' perceptions of the professional role. *Physical Therapy, 67*(2), 226–233.

Coren, A., Andreassi, M., Blood, H., & Kent, B. (1987). Factors relating to physical therapy students' decisions to work with elderly patients. *Physical Therapy, 67*(1), 60–65.

Deitz, J. C., Crowe, T. K., & Harris, S. R. (1987). Relationship between infant neuromotor assessment and preschool motor measures. *Physical Therapy, 67*(1), 14–17.

Gogia, P. P., Braatz, J. H., Rose, S. J., & Norton, B. J. (1987). Reliability and validity of goniometric measurements at the knee. *Physical Therapy, 67*(2), 192–195.

Graham, W. G., & Bradley, D. A. (1978). Efficacy of chest physiotherapy and intermittent positive pressure breathing in the resolution of pneumonia. *New England Journal of Medicine, 229*, 624–627.

Hamilton-Dodd, C., Kawamoto, T., Clark, F., Burke, J. P., & Fanchiang, S. P. (1989). The effects of a maternal preparation program on mother-infant pairs: A pilot study. *American Journal of Occupational Therapy, 43*(8), 513–521.

Hasselkus, B. R., & Safrit, M. J. (1976). Measurement in occupational therapy. *American Journal of Occupational Therapy, 30*(7), 429–436.

Liu, H., Currier, D. P., & Threlkeld, A. J. (1987). Circulatory response of digital arteries associated with electrical stimulation of calf muscle in healthy subjects. *Physical Therapy, 67*(3), 340–345.

Lohmann, K. N., Rayhel, H. E., Schneiderwind, W. P., & Danoff, J. V. (1987). Static measurement of tibia vara. *Physical Therapy, 67*(2), 196–199.

Magalhaes, L., Koomar, J., & Cermak, S. (1989). Bilateral motor coordination in 5- to 9-year-old children: A pilot study. *American Journal of Occupational Therapy, 43*(7), 437–443.

Mitchell, M. J., Daines, G. E., & Thomas, B. L. (1987). Effect of L-tryptophan and phenylalanine on burning pain threshold. *Physical Therapy, 67*(2), 203–205.

Moncur, C. (1987). Perceptions of physical therapy competencies in rheumatology. *Physical Therapy, 67*(3), 331–339.

Oyster, C. K., Hanten, W. P., & Llorens, L. S. (1987). *Introduction to research: A guide for the health science professional*. Philadelphia: J.B. Lippincott.

Partridge, C. J., & Barnitt, R. E. (1986). *Research guidelines: A handbook for therapists*. Rockville, MD: Aspen Publishers.

Schaefer, R. L., & Anderson, R. B. (1989). *The student edition of Minitab: Statistical software adapted for education*. Reading, MA: Addison-Wesley Publishing and Benjamin/Cummings Publishing.

Shinabarger, N. I. (1987). Limited joint mobility in adults with diabetes mellitus. *Physical Therapy, 67*(2), 215–218.

Taylor, K., Newton. R. A., Personius, W. J., & Bush, R. M. (1987). Effects of interferential current stimulation for treatment of subjects with recurrent jaw pain. *Physical Therapy, 67*(3), 346–350.

ADDITIONAL READING

Ethridge, D., & McSweeney, M. (1971). Research in occupational therapy: 5. Data interpretation, results and conclusions. *American Journal of Occupational Therapy*, XXV(3), 149–154.

Greenstein, L. R. (1980). Teaching research: An introduction to statistical concepts and research terminology. *American Journal of Occupational Therapy, 34*(5), 320–327.

Kerlinger, F. N. (1973). *Foundations of behavioral research*. New York: Holt, Rinehart & Winston.

Koosis, D. (1985). *Statistics: A self-teaching guide*. New York: John Wiley & Sons.

Lee, E. S., Forthofer, R. N., & Lorimer, R. J. (1989). *Analyzing complex survey data*. No. 71 in Quantitative Applications in the Social Sciences Series. Newbury Park, CA: Sage Publications.

Lodge, M. (1981). *Magnitude scaling: Quantitative measurement of opinions*. No. 25 in Quantitative Applications in the Social Sciences Series. Newbury Park, CA: Sage Publications.

Mainland, D. (1969). Statistical ward rounds 17 & 18: Some research terms for beginners: definitions, components and examples. *Clinical Pharmacological Therapy, 10*, 714–736.

Reynolds, H. T. (1984). *Analysis of nominal data*. No. 7 in Quantitative Applications in the Social Sciences Series. Newbury Park, CA: Sage Publications.

Rowntree, D. (1981). *Statistics without tears: A primer for non-mathematicians*. New York: Charles Scribner's Sons.

9

Final Preparation before Implementing the Research Plan

At this point, you are almost ready to conduct your project. There are just two more items that need to be dealt with before you begin. First, permission must be gained from the relevant human subjects committee(s) to put your study into practice, and second, you should consider running a pilot study.

HUMAN SUBJECTS COMMITTEE PROCEDURES

Before you can begin to carry out your research project, you must submit a proposal describing your study to the human subjects committee responsible for safeguarding the rights of the subjects you will be using. If you are a student, there will be a committee within the university; if you are a therapist, there will be a committee within or connected to your facility. Students planning to study patients will frequently need to gain consent from the human subjects committees of both the university and the treating facility. (These committees may be known by other names, such as institutional review board or research protocol review committee.)

The purpose of human subjects committees is to ensure that individuals participating as subjects in research studies are protected and that ethical research standards are being employed. This concern for the welfare of human subjects in medical research studies was not organized or systematized worldwide until 1964, when the 18th World Medical Assembly was held in Helsinki, Finland. At that meeting, what has come to be known as the Declaration of Helsinki was adopted by the assembly and has since provided the guiding principles for human subject research. The Declaration of Helsinki is reprinted in Appendix G.

Before embarking on your study, you must present a proposal to the appropriate human subjects committee(s) outlining the purpose, hypotheses, background, definitions of terms, and methodology of the study, together with procedures you will use to ensure the safety of the subjects. When committee members are satisfied that their requirements have been met, they will give permission to go ahead with the research study. The committee will review the proposal to see if it meets the following criteria:

1. The scientific logic upon which the study is constructed is sound.
2. The study is worthwhile.
3. The proposed methodology is sound.
4. Procedures are safe.
5. The investigator has the skills to perform the study.
6. There is provision for informed consent by subjects.
7. The benefits of participating in the study outweigh the risks.
8. Subjects may withdraw their consent to participate at any time.
9. Subjects' confidentiality will be protected.
10. Necessary treatment will not be withheld.

To review these items in more detail: (1) The first issue will be addressed by the material you present to the committee on the background, literature review, and scope of the study. These sections of the proposal have already been prepared from the work you did in Chapters 2, 3, and 6, and a summary of these sections will explain the scientific logic of the study to the committee. (2) The second issue, that the study is worthwhile, can be answered by a summary of the sections you prepared on the purpose and significance of the study, following Chapter 3. (3) and (4) The soundness of the proposed methodology will be addressed by the material in Chapters 5 to 8 containing the research design and method of collecting and analyzing data. The committee will decide whether the method is appropriate to the study and whether it will achieve the purpose of the study.

Stein (1989, p. 52) has presented a useful diagram showing the purposes of experimental research and containing the logical flow of material for which a committee will be looking. The diagram is presented in Figure 9-1 with minor modifications.

(5) Your qualifications for conducting the research may be substantiated by submission of a resumé or by your presence before the committee to present your credentials.

(6) Gaining informed consent means that subjects must understand the nature of the project, what procedures will be used, and to what use the results will be put. In survey research, if subjects return the survey, they have given their tacit consent to participate in the study. In experimental and quasi-experimental studies, subjects give their consent in writing, before a witness, and must be offered a copy of the form they have signed. A sample of an informed consent form is given in Appendix H.

If you feel a subject is unable to give informed consent by virtue of cognitive or physical incapacity or age, the consent of the legal guardian must be obtained. Any explanation of the study must be stated in lay terms. If the subjects are children, the consent of the parents or guardians must be obtained (see Appendix H). If the nature of the research dictates that you cannot tell subjects the purpose of the study (because the knowledge might bias results/responses), that must be explained honestly.

(7) In the consent form, any risks or benefits that may result from participating in the study must be explained to subjects (see Appendix H). The committee will expect that the

Purpose	To observe cause-effect relationships in animals	To analyze human processes in normal subjects	To compare effectiveness of treatment methods for disabled subjects
Significance	Implications for understanding disease processes	Implications for discovering general laws of human physiological and motoric responses	Implications for justifying new treatment techniques

Figure 9-1 Justifying research.

benefits will outweigh the risks. Possible side effects of the study should be pointed out, and precautions that will be taken by the researcher to prevent damage to subjects should be discussed. The place and length of time for the study sessions should be explained (see Appendix H).

(8) Included in the informed consent form should be a statement that there will be no reprisal regardless of the subject's willingness to participate. Occasionally, clients may fear that their treatment may be compromised in some way if they refuse to participate in a study — perhaps they feel they will not receive the same quality care as the study participants. This is a problem especially if the therapist carrying out the study is also the clients' treating therapist. It must also be made clear in the written consent form that subjects can terminate participation in the study at any point without fear of reprisal (see Appendix H).

(9) If there has been any type of recording of subjects' behavior or output (such as audio or videotape recording) or samples of subjects' writing, drawings, or paintings, the document must state how these materials will be used and what will happen to them at the conclusion of the study. It is usual to offer subjects and/or their guardians an opportunity to view the materials if they wish. Subjects must be assured that materials will be kept in a secure place during the study, and must be told who will have access to them (see Appendices H and I).

If the results of the study are to be published, subjects need to know that their anonymity is guaranteed. Separate written permission must be gained if photographs are to be used in the published material (see Appendix I).

Survey respondents also need to be assured that their anonymity will be guarded. This is usually accomplished by having them return the surveys anonymously. Survey respondents are not asked to sign a consent form, because responding to the survey is seen in itself as consent to participate.

If subjects are to be paid for their participation in the study, payment should be based on work and time considerations rather than as compensation for any risk involved or as inducement to poor subjects to participate.

(10) Finally, there is the issue of withholding treatment. If there are to be experimental and control groups in the study, subjects might not be told to which group they are assigned. If the study is conducted to test a new procedure with the experimental group, the control group may either receive the standard treatment or no treatment. Some facilities will not permit subjects to be in control groups that do not receive treatment, which is understandable, because they are generally in the facility for the express purpose of being treated. This expectation will dictate the activity of the control group, and investigators must abide by the facility's regulations.

ETHICS

As well as meeting the demands of human subjects committees, researchers are expected to behave ethically in all areas of their practice. It is the responsibility of the investigators themselves to know the rules of conduct. Researchers are expected to show integrity and to be guided by ethical principles that include respecting the rights of subjects, abiding by the research design, and reporting results as they are found.

It is particularly important to guard zealously the rights of subjects who are in institutional environments such as facilities for the mentally retarded, mental hospitals, and prisons. People in these settings are especially vulnerable and are not usually in a position to serve as their own advocates; researchers must be especially careful not to take advantage of them.

Another ethical consideration is that investigators must abide by the research design as it was presented to and approved by the human subjects committee. Unexpected issues may arise that cause researchers to redesign their study. If this is the case, the revised design must be submitted to the committee to ensure that it still meets requirements. If any of the changes affects the agreement signed by the subjects, they too must be informed and a new agreement signed.

Finally, there are definite ethical standards involving the reporting of research results. Sometimes the results are such that some findings support the hypotheses while others do not. All findings must be reported. If findings are not at the identified level for statistical significance, they must be presented as found. The highest integrity must be maintained in reporting on all phases of the study, exactly as they occurred.

PILOT STUDIES

Several times throughout this book a pilot study has been suggested as a way to check on the feasibility of various components of the project. We now examine what a pilot study should comprise, how it is done, and what can be learned from it.

The pilot study is a preliminary trial of the study or a ministudy and should be performed at some point before the final study. Most of the steps of the final study should be included in the pilot study, but on a smaller scale. Subjects for the pilot should be selected from the target population so that results are likely to be representative of what will happen in the final study. The number of subjects used will be considerably smaller than the final sample size. The process will be that which is proposed for the major study, even including analysis of the data generated from the pilot group. As a result, the pilot study provides an evaluation of the proposed process and may be used to remove flaws.

Sometimes problems are found in the logic that leads to the hypotheses, in which case a major revision of the research questions may be in order. At other times, simple changes in the measuring instrument or subject selection criteria may be sufficient to make the project satisfactory. Some modifications of the original proposal are almost always necessary, so pilot studies invariably improve the design and data of the final projects. It is always worthwhile to take the time and effort to perform a pilot study.

The items that may be tested for feasibility in a pilot study concern either methodology or scientific logic. Those concerning scientific logic might include such items as:

- Whether the problem being studied has been too broadly or too narrowly defined
- Whether or not the variables selected were suitable
- Whether the resulting data will address the purpose of the study

Whereas methodological issues might include:

- Whether or not survey questions are clearly stated and unambiguous
- Whether or not the investigative methods generate information suitable for answering the research question
- The availability of appropriate subjects
- That the variables are discrete and can be measured meaningfully
- Whether or not the measuring instrument is accurate and practical

Typically, there are certain items in each type of research design that can be best evaluated by a pilot study. For example, in survey research the manner in which questions are composed is all-important. The investigator wishes to know if respondents understand the meaning of questions, if questions elicit the type of information desired, and if the survey is too long or too short. Respondents should know that they are answering a pilot study instrument and that they will be asked for suggestions for improvements in the questionnaire and/or cover letter and how long it took them to complete the survey.

In performing experimental research, it may be difficult to perform a pilot study because the investigator may have access to only a few subjects who meet the selection criteria. If subjects are used for a pilot study, there may not be sufficient subjects for the final study. In behavioral research, it is often the case that subjects cannot be used twice—once in the pilot study and again in the final study—because the effects of the pilot treatment may influence the results of the final study treatment. It is sometimes possible to deal with this problem by using a pilot sample of suitable individuals from another facility or by using a slightly different population. This solution is often preferable to eliminating the pilot altogether.

Sometimes true experimental and quasi-experimental research studies are performed on such small samples that they constitute pilot studies rather than true studies. Because there has been no pilot study, researchers occasionally undertake these studies with uncertain methodology and unclear justification for the study. When the results of such projects are published, inevitably there is a list of limitations and disclaimers at the end of the report. The investigator should have regarded the project as a pilot study, then pursued a second study, amending philosophy and procedures based on the limitations of the first. This would make the results of the second study more valid, meaningful, and publishable (see Boxes 9–A and 9–B).

Case study research is often conducted as a pilot study, in the sense that the individual case is used to generate hypotheses that will later be tested in an experimental manner on a large sample of similar subjects. However, if the investigator does not intend the case study to be a pilot for a larger study, some portions of the study may be piloted ahead of time. Portions that may be pre-tested include such things as the use of equipment, the validity of a measuring instrument, or the usefulness of a data-gathering technique.

Historical research does not lend itself to the use of a single pilot study, since there is one event or chain of events being studied; if an unsatisfactory method of data collection has been used, no harm has been done to the event and other methods may be explored. Generally, it is considered part of the study methodology to try different forms of data collection and data analysis until satisfactory methods are found.

Ethnographic research is similar to historical research in this respect. There is one culture or program under study, and data can be collected and analyzed in many ways until the process is considered satisfactory. Sometimes an event within the culture or treatment program will occur only once (such as an unusual ceremony or a patient trying a rare treatment), and in that case the investigator must be ready with the best methodology to capture that event at the moment it occurs. This may require preparation by testing certain techniques ahead of time — in other words, running a pilot study — perhaps in a simulated situation. It is almost always methodology, rather than scientific logic or philosophical issues, that needs to be tested in this type of once-only research. In fact in ethnographic research, proposing and rejecting philosophical issues in the data analysis is one of the main ways of interpreting data, as was described in the section on pattern matching, explanation building, and triangulation (see Chapter 7).

In methodological research, the pilot study is built into the research process at the stage when the newly developed measure is tested on a sample, when changes are made, and when the revised measure is tested again. The process may occur several times before the researcher feels satisfied with the results. This test/retest procedure serves the same purpose as a pilot study and may be considered as such.

In the summative component of evaluation research, the survey instruments used to garner data about the program under study may appropriately be subjected to a pilot study. The reasons and procedures for doing so will be similar to those mentioned under survey

---

Box 9–A

"In a dental study conducted several years ago, the first batches of data collected were incomplete and ratings were remarkably similar across patients. The problem was that dental hygienists who were collecting the data had not been included in the decision-making process and did not appreciate data collection requirements. Piloting in that case should have included not only a sample of patients similar to the proposed subjects, but a sample of dental hygienists similar to those who would be collecting data. In the end, the inadequate data had to be treated as a pilot and discarded [from the final study]."
(Grady & Strudler Wallston, 1988, p. 148)

> **Box 9–B**
>
> In discussing the design of qualitative research, Marshall and Rossman (1989) state that:
>
> . . . use of a pilot can lend credence to the researcher's claim that he can conduct such a study. He can illustrate his ability to manage qualitative research by describing initial observations or interviews. . . . A description of initial observations demonstrates not only the ability to manage this research, but also the strength of the approach for revealing enticing research questions. Inclusion of a description of a pilot study or initial observations can strengthen the proposal.
>
> (p. 51)

research, namely, to ensure that the questions will elicit needed data and will be understood by respondents.

Finally, one very important purpose for performing a pilot study is that it gives you a chance to practice conducting research. Like most things, research becomes easier and improves in quality the more often it is practiced. A pilot study gives the novice researcher a good opportunity to gain skill while achieving the all-important goal of improving the research design.

IMPLEMENTING THE PROJECT

You are finally ready to carry out your research project. As you can see, it takes an enormous amount of work to be ready to actually conduct the treatment/action component of a research study. Yet often, this is the only component that people equate with the term *research*.

There are now the practical issues to be arranged. Depending on the type of research, these may be as varied as setting up times and places to meet with subjects, arranging access to rooms and equipment, training raters or other participants in the study, copying and mailing surveys, locating suitable client records for review, or arranging to videotape a group procedure.

STUMBLING BLOCKS

Investigators often underestimate the length of time needed to gain permission from a human subjects committee. This process can take anywhere from 1 to 4 months, depending on how frequently the committee meets and whether all materials have been submitted correctly and completely. If there are components of the protocol that need to be revised, it may take even longer. The investigator should probably submit the proposal to the committee at about the time that the research protocol is being written (by the end of the procedures in Chapter 5). This should allow sufficient time for notification by the committee prior to the start of data collection.

Much time and aggravation can be saved by finding out ahead of time the exact requirements of the committee to which you are applying, because they vary. Some committees have detailed written instructions, while others merely give a verbal outline. The packet of instructions for the Harvard Committee on Human Studies (1975), for instance, is about 30 pages long, while the submission requirements for a day activity program with which I am familiar are not defined in writing at all. A sample of guidelines for informed consent for a children's hospital is given in Appendix J.

It is strongly recommended that you take the time to locate the administrator of the human subjects committee and get to know this person on a first-name basis. It is then likely that you will be informed of exact requirements or of any changes in plans (such as meeting dates) and that your material will be processed in a timely fashion.

When describing your study to potential subjects in order to obtain their consent to participate, it is sometimes difficult to know if the explanation has been fully understood. This may be especially true when talking to mentally retarded or mentally ill clients. If there is any doubt about the client's comprehension, it is a good idea to have present the person who knows the client best, to assess how much is understood and perhaps to reword the explanation so that it is meaningful to the client. Some human subjects committees require that a member of the committee be present on such an occasion, while others have a human rights officer who will serve this purpose.

WORKSHEETS

PROPOSAL FOR HUMAN SUBJECTS COMMITTEE

Find out which human subjects committee is responsible for the population you are intending to study. Request a copy of that committee's requirements. Following the guidelines, prepare a proposal to present to the committee. The committee may want the following information in one format or another:

1. A general description of your study, including its *background*. Detail the *problem* you will be addressing and your *purpose* (what you hope to achieve). *Define the terms* you will be using and spell out the *hypotheses*. You should state the importance or *significance* of the project. Describe the *methodology* you will use; include subjects, research design, and data collection methods. All of this material is available from the worksheets in previous chapters.

2. Provide the informed consent statement you will present to subjects for their signature (see sample in Appendix H). Remember to:

- Include the purpose of the study.
- Include the place and the amount of time the study will require of subjects.
- Include a description of the procedure to be used.
- State that participation is voluntary.
- State that participation can be withdrawn at any time without fear or reprisal.
- List the risks and benefits of the study.
- Cite any costs that may be involved.
- Describe how confidentiality will be protected.
- Give the name of someone who will be available to answer questions on the research.
- State that a copy of this statement will be offered to subjects.
- Provide a space for the subjects' signature, a witness's signature, and if needed, a parent/guardian signature.
- Provide a space for the date of the signatures.

    Prepare an informed consent statement.

State the names of all the investigators involved in the study, list your qualifications as head of the research team, and state why you are qualified to carry out the proposed research project:

After this material is written, put it into an organized packet, and send it to the human subjects committee in time for the next meeting. Find out if you may be present at the meeting in order to answer questions about your proposal. Find out when and in what manner you will be advised if your proposal is accepted.

PILOT STUDY

Decide if your study lends itself to a pilot study. Will methodological issues or scientific logic issues, or both, need to be piloted? List the parts you think could be improved by a pilot study:

Methodological issues:

Scientific logic issues:

Can you afford to use some of the target population for the pilot study sample?

If so, how will you select them?

Write a protocol for a pilot study. Remember that it will resemble the protocol you wrote for the study itself (see Worksheets following Chapter 5):

Subject criteria

Selection method

Hypotheses

Dependent and independent variables

Procedures for treatment

Procedures for observation

Data collection methods

Data analysis methods

REFERENCES

Grady, K. E., & Strudler Wallston, B. (1988). *Research in health care settings*. No. 14 in Applied Social Research Methods Series. Newbury Park, CA: Sage Publications.

The Harvard Committee on Human Studies. (1975). *Policies and procedures of the Harvard Committee on Human Studies:* Policies and procedures governing the conduct of research, development, or related activities involving human subjects carried out at the Harvard Medical School or Harvard School of Dental Medicine or under their aegis in the facilities of an affiliated institution. Cambridge, MA: Harvard Medical School and Harvard School of Dental Medicine.

Marshall, C., & Rossman, G. B. (1989). *Designing qualitative research*. Newbury Park, CA: Sage Publications.

Stein, F. (1989). *Anatomy of clinical research: An introduction to scientific inquiry in medicine, rehabilitation and related health professions*. Thorofare, NJ: Slack, Inc.

ADDITIONAL READING

American Occupational Therapy Foundation: Research Advisory Council. (1986). *Ethical considerations for research in occupational therapy*. Rockville, MD: Author.

Berger, R. M., & Patchner, M. A. (1988). Chapter 7: Research ethics. In *Implementing the research plan: A guide for the helping professions* (pp. 143–154). No. 51 in Human Services Guides Series. Newbury Park, CA: Sage Publications.

Haywood, H. C. (1976). The ethics of doing research . . . and of not doing it. *American Journal of Mental Deficiency, 81*(4), 311–317.

Michels, E. (1976). Research and human rights, 2. *Physical Therapy, 56*, 546–550.

Noonan, M. J., & Bickel, W. K. (1981). The ethics of experimental designs. *Mental Retardation, 19*(6), 271–274.

Schwartzberg, S. L. (1980). The Foundation: Issues in human subject occupational therapy research. *American Journal of Occupational Therapy, 34*(8), 537–538.

10

Reporting Results and Drawing Conclusions

Now that you have conducted the study and gathered information about your subjects, you need to analyze the data using the quantitative or qualitative analysis methods that you planned earlier. This chapter will discuss the presentation of your results, how to display data pictorially, how to approach the interpretations and conclusions section, and the content of the summary section.

PRESENTATION OF RESULTS

In the results section of a paper, only the facts of the study are presented, with no interpretation. Authors must be careful not to include their own biases or conclusions in the results section. Rather they must keep to a factual recording of what actually happened and what was actually found.

All the results must be mentioned in the results section of a report — not solely the ones that substantiate the hypotheses or suit the investigator's needs. Even though you later will present your own interpretations and conclusions from the results, readers must be able to decide for themselves the efficacy of these conclusions by having all the data at hand. At the end of the results section, it should be clearly stated which of the hypotheses were or were not supported. In the case of inferential statistical results, the reader should be told if the significance level established at the start of the project was reached.

First you need to describe the subjects in a numerical manner. You will offer such information as: 75 percent of the sample were older than 50 years of age, and the age range of the entire group was from 30 years to 60 years. Or: "Thirty undergraduate students not studying occupational therapy or physical therapy (15 males, 15 females) with a mean age of 19.0 years participated in the study" (Steinbeck, 1986, p. 531). From this type of information, it will be possible for readers to gain a clear picture of the study sample, so that later they may superimpose the findings of the study on that picture.

No matter what type of research design you have used, you will want to describe the sample. It is usual to present frequencies, percentages, a range, and some sort of central tendency (such as the mean) for the data. This information will give readers solid information about what your subjects looked like and how they performed in the study (see Box 10–A).

Box 10-A

Schwartzberg (1982) spent considerable time delineating her sample in a descriptive study yielding qualitative data concerning psychiatric patients' perceptions of what facilitates or blocks their occupational performance. She describes their age (n, range), gender (n), marital status (%, n), number of children (n, mean), religion (n, ratio), occupation (n, ratio), educational level (n, %, mean), number of psychiatric hospitalizations (n, %, ratio), psychopharmacological status (n, %), and diagnosis (n, ratio). Because this descriptive study used patients' self-report for data (via interview), it was essential for the reader to have detailed information about those patients in order to put what was said into context and to make comparisons with other patients.

REPORTING QUANTITATIVE DATA

If you have conducted experimental, quasi-experimental, or correlational research, your study will probably have yielded quantitative data, and you will be using statistical procedures to determine if there are meaningful differences or similarities between groups. The probability ratios will provide that information and will indicate if the hypotheses have been substantiated. At this point, go back to each of the hypotheses and check them against the statistical results (see Box 10-B). For each hypothesis, inform readers if the hypothesis was substantiated, give the probability level, then report the details of the findings. It is customary for results to be reported from the general to the specific.

REPORTING QUALITATIVE DATA

If you have conducted survey, historical, or ethnographic research, you will probably have garnered non-quantitative or qualitative data. The data will continue to be reported in a manner similar to that used to describe the sample, that is, using frequencies, percentages, ranges, and central tendencies.

In a descriptive study reporting on the incidence of upper extremity discomfort among piano students, Revak (1989) reports the results as shown in Box 10-C. This particular study used a survey to generate data; therefore, all the results lend themselves to being described in a similar style. Thus, Revak describes the results concerning the respondents' discomfort as shown in Box 10-D. The author continues to report the results in this fashion, listing frequencies and percentages for each finding in the study so that readers gain a graphic picture of the pianist respondents and their upper extremity discomforts. This is a typical and most effective method for reporting descriptive research findings. Having such a complete roster of data about respondents allows readers to form their own opinions and draw their own conclusions concerning the sample.

Box 10-B

A study was conducted comparing younger subjects (aged 20 to 60 years) with older subjects (aged 61 to 80 years) on body image, as measured by a semantic differential scale of attitudes toward various body parts (Van Deusen, Harlowe, & Baker, 1989). Therapists subjected data from the two groups to the Mann-Whitney U Test to test the hypotheses that elderly and younger adults would have significantly different perceptions of their trunk, arms, hands, and legs. The level of significance was set at $p < .05$. The study showed that elderly subjects perceive only their hands as substantially different from those of younger adults.

To determine in which direction the difference lay, the investigators turned to the means of scores on the semantic differential. They found that the mean for the older group was smaller (less positive) for hands than the mean for the younger group, thus they had a finding: that community-based elders had a less positive body image regarding their hands than did younger adults.

Box 10–C

"Seventy-one students, or 31% of the survey sample, returned their questionnaires. The highest response rate (89%) from an individual school was obtained from the only school that permitted direct mailings to the students. Although two-thirds of the total number of students surveyed were enrolled in one of two universities, only 20% of the questionnaires distributed to those students were returned. . . .

"The majority (75%) of respondents were undergraduates. Sixty-eight percent of the respondents were women, and 32% were men. . . .

"Thirty (42%) of the respondents indicated that they had experienced physical discomfort in their hands or arms that persisted or recurred for more than 1 week and that impaired their ability to practice the piano. The respondents with physical discomfort in their upper extremities were predominantly women (86%), under 25 years of age (70%), and right-hand dominant (75%). Although female respondents out-numbered male respondents by a ratio of 2:1, women appeared to have a greater incidence of physical discomfort in their upper extremities than men did."

(Revak, 1989, pp. 150–151)

You may have subjected the data to one or more of the coding procedures. The results of the coding must be presented as clearly and simply as possible. In this type of presentation, it is the weight of the evidence that will determine if the hypotheses have been substantiated — a judgment the investigator must make, because it is not possible to subject the evidence to statistical significance testing (see Box 10–E).

PICTORIAL DISPLAY OF DATA

Sometimes it is useful to display data pictorially. This allows readers to gain an immediate and overall concept of the results and lets them make sense of quantities of data at a glance; as the old saying goes, "A picture is worth a thousand words" — or, in this case, a thousand numbers. The use of tables, graphs, or charts can eliminate many complicated or boring sentences but they should be used judiciously — too many become confusing.

There are many pictorial means for presenting data. The following are some of the most commonly used. Simple lists of frequencies and percentages are probably best presented in tabular form. Use tables to consolidate and present data, such as numbers of pounds squeezed on a goniometer. If scores were arranged in order from highest to lowest (rank ordering), for example, readers could easily gain an overview of a group of responses.

Box 10–D

"Eighty-three percent of the respondents with physical discomfort reported more than one symptom. Pain or aching of the upper extremities was the predominant discomfort experienced (see Table 1). . . .

"The respondents were divided into two groups, those who sought treatment and those who did not. The discomforts reported by each group differed. Pain/aching (82%) was the only physical discomfort reported by more than half of the students who sought medical treatment. Students in this group also frequently complained of tenderness (47%). Over half of the students not seeking medical treatment reported pain/aching (71%), fatigue (65%), weakness (59%), and muscle cramp (53%). . . .

"Fifteen (50%) of the students that experienced physical discomfort reported it in both hands and/or arms. Eight students reported discomfort only on the right side, and six students reported discomfort only on the left. As shown in Table 2, the most frequent regions of discomfort were the hand (49%), the forearm (19%), and the wrist (16%). Discomfort was reported nearly equally on the dorsal and volar surfaces of the wrist and forearm."

(Revak, 1989, pp. 150–151)

Box 10-E

Schwartzberg (1982) used thematic coding in a study seeking to learn, directly from hospitalized psychiatric patients, what facilitates or blocks performance of activities of daily living. Informants were interviewed with a set of open-ended questions, and the interview transcripts were thematically analyzed. The thematic analysis led to inferences about what facilitated or blocked occupational performance. The results section occupied a large portion of the article and reported 11 inferences gleaned from the thematic coding, each presented with selected excerpts from informant interviews.

They could see the range of scores; the highest, lowest, and middle scores; and could compare one person's scores against the others. Table 10-1 shows the rank ordering of two types of values reported by 385 occupational therapy administrators and clinicians.

Tables are especially useful for condensing large quantities of data so that the reader can make sense of the information more readily. Suppose a study yielded 50 scores of degrees of elbow flexion for a group of patients. Even presenting the 50 scores in order of magnitude would be difficult for a reader to digest and think about usefully. In this case, grouping the scores, say into units of 20, would reduce the data and allow the reader to grasp its implications more efficiently (Table 10-2). From this table it is possible to quickly understand the spread of scores; that most patients had flexion in the midrange ($60°-120°$), while few patients had flexion at the greater and smaller angles. Even though some detail is lost in this type of grouping, it is generally a useful and efficient representation of data.

Tables are commonly used to illustrate the findings from descriptive and inferential statistics. In this case, they can present detailed materials more easily and in less space

Table 10-1

Rank Ordering of Terminal and Instrumental Values by Occupational Therapy Administrators and Clinicians (N = 385)

	Administrators' Rank Ordering (n = 201)	Clinicians' Rank Ordering (n = 184)	Total Group Rank Ordering
Terminal values:			
Self-respect	1	2	2
Health	2	1	1
A sense of accomplishment	3	5	4
Inner harmony	4	3	3
Freedom	5	6	5
Wisdom	6	4	6
Mature love	7	7	7
An exciting life	8	8	8
A comfortable life	9	9	9
Equality	10	10	10
Social recognition	11	12	12
Pleasure	12	11	11
Instrumental values:			
Capable	1	3	3
Honest	2	1	1
Responsible	3	2	2
Independent	4	4	4
Loving	5	5	5
Helpful	6	6	6
Courageous	7	9	9
Broad-minded	8	7	7
Loyal	9	8	8
Imaginative	10	10	10
Ambitious	11	11	11
Obedient	12	12	12

Table 10–2
Degrees of Elbow Flexion Following Treatment (n = 50)

Degrees of Elbow Flexion	Frequency of Occurrence
20–40	2
40–60	4
60–80	9
80–100	10
100–120	12
120–140	9
140–160	3
160–180	1

than would be required by narration. It is not necessary to repeat all the table data in the text; the investigator should merely highlight important points. Tables 10–3 and 10–4 present data generated from descriptive statistics and inferential statistics.

While tables are invaluable for communicating concisely a large set of numbers, many people find it difficult to get the "big picture" from a table. This is why we turn to graphs to convey a visual image of a distribution of items or events, or changes in numbers of items over time, or how several items compare.

There are many types of graphs, one of the most popular being the frequency polygon, illustrated in Figure 10–1, where a single line joins frequency points of occurrence. There is traditionally a y-axis noting the frequency of items or events and an x-axis charting the

Table 10–3
Distribution of Demographic Characteristics for Occupational Therapy Administrators and Clinicians (N = 385)

Demographic Characteristic	Administrators (n = 201)		Clinicians (n = 184)		Total group	
	Frequency	Percent	Frequency	Percent	Frequency	Percent
Age:						
20–25 years	0	0	2	1	2	0.5
26–30 years	17	9	46	25	63	16
31–35 years	56	28	52	28	108	28
36–40 years	33	16	26	14	59	15
41–50 years	53	26	40	22	93	24
51+ years	42	21	18	10	60	16
College degrees:						
BA or BS in OT	95	47	113	61	208	57
Certification in OT	13	10	17	9	30	8
MOT	10	6	8	4	18	6
MA or MS in OT	21	11	4	2	25	7
Non-OT MA/MS	47	25	19	15	66	17
Doctorate	4	2	0	0	4	1
When subject decided to become an OT:						
Jr. high school	20	10	11	6	31	8
Sr. high school	60	30	61	33	121	31
First 2 yrs. of college	80	40	71	39	151	39
Second 2 yrs. of college	18	9	16	9	34	9
After college	12	6	14	8	26	7
Other	11	5	11	6	22	6
Age when took first job as an OT:						
20–25 years	178	89	156	85	334	87
26–30 years	14	7	14	8	28	7
31–35 years	4	2	5	3	9	2
36–40 years	2	1	5	3	7	2
41+ years	5	2	4	2	9	2
Specialty within OT:						
Psychiatry	60	30	49	27	109	29
Pediatrics	31	15	59	32	90	24
Physical disabilities	95	47	63	35	158	41
Geriatrics	15	8	11	6	26	7

Table 10-4
Differences Between Administrators and Clinicians on Demographic Characteristics (N = 385)

Role by Characteristic	Pearson Chi-square	Significance Level
Role by age	31.22	0.00*
Role by degree	31.22	0.00*
Role by age when decided to become an OT	2.68	0.75
Role by age at taking first job	2.24	0.69
Role by specialty in OT	18.20	0.00*
Role by mother's education	3.71	0.81
Role by father's education	7.73	0.36
Role by mentor	6.22	0.10

*$p < .001$

item under study. In Figure 10-1, the percentages of time when a patient was free from restraint are entered on the graph. All of the points are joined to form a continuous line on the graph. The bar graph or histogram is illustrated in Figure 10-2 and is similar to the frequency polygon, except that it is formed by drawing a vertical bar at each frequency gained, across the width of the score interval. The number of students achieving each test score form a solid block on the graph; in this way, the histogram offers a strong visual impact.

When one group of scores is compared against another, such as scores from 1989 and scores from 1990, both types of graph may be used, but the histogram is particularly visually effective. Figures 10-3 and 10-4 illustrate this point.

A pie chart is often used to depict a breakdown of some quantity, for example, expenditures for a program or types of employees in a facility, as shown in Figure 10-5.

These are just three of the many possibilities for displaying data pictorially. For further ideas, you may refer to the books mentioned in the Additional Reading list at the end of this chapter.

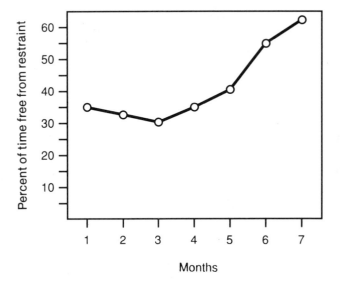

Figure 10-1 Percent of time per month free from restraint. (From Bright, T., Bittick, K., & Fleeman, B. [1981]. Reduction of self-injurious behavior using sensory integrative techniques. *American Journal of Occupational Therapy, 35* [3], 167-172. Copyright 1981. Reprinted with permission.)

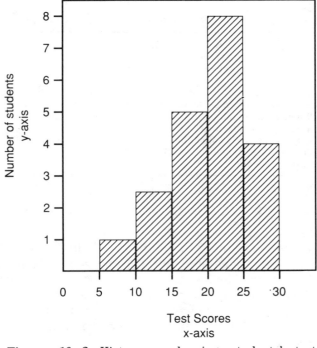

Figure 10-2 Histogram showing students' test scores.

If you use pictorial methods for presenting data, be sure to refer to specific tables or figures in the text. Label them correctly—tables are called "tables," while graphs, charts, drawings, photographs, and so forth, are called "figures." In the text, tell readers what to look for in the tables and figures, picking out salient features. You do not need to repeat all the material shown in the pictorial, but you should highlight the most important points.

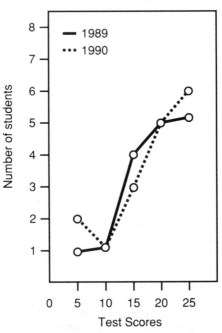

Figure 10-3 Polygon showing students' test scores for 1989 and 1990.

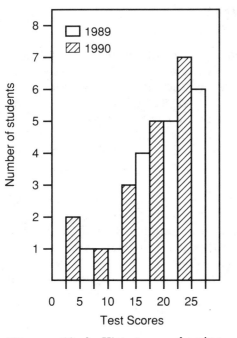

Figure 10-4 Histogram showing students' test scores for 1989 and 1990.

With accurate and complete titles, column headings, axes labels, and footnotes, tables should be understandable on their own, without text. Titles should be concise and describe exactly the information included. If a table were to be studied without any text, the title should be complete enough for readers to know what to expect and to be able to read the contents.

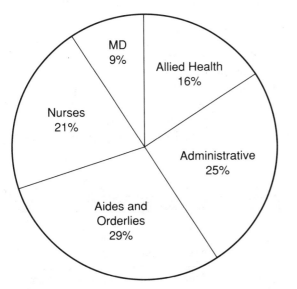

Figure 10-5 Pie chart depicting percentages of personnel employed in a hospital.

INTERPRETATIONS AND CONCLUSIONS

Now go back to the literature review. It is time to compare your results with those of others who have studied the topic. Integrate your findings with those of previous studies, and note points of agreement and departure. You might have suggestions as to why you found different results, as pointed out by the authors in the study described in Box 10-F. The purpose of comparing your findings with those of similar studies is to put your study in a context with work that has already been done on the topic. Ideally, your study should be contributing to a larger body of work—adding one more brick to the wall of knowledge about that topic—perhaps adding evidence that will tip the scales in one direction or the other concerning theory about a particular issue.

At this point, you may speculate and draw your own conclusions about what the results mean. You are interpreting the results. Start by discussing the similarities and differences between the results of your study and those of other studies. Keep adding to the reader's understanding of the entire problem under investigation with each new statement you make, relating your findings to other people's theories about the problem. Any finding is fair game for comment, as long as it was reported in the results section. However, you should not discuss a finding that was not reported. This is also true of theorists. If an author was not mentioned in the literature review section, that person's name may not be introduced in the conclusion section.

Findings that do not support the hypotheses or do not conform with other findings from the study should be commented upon. It is customary to speculate as to why they occurred and what they might mean, as shown in Box 10-G. Notice the author does not apologize for the fact that the finding does not conclusively support the hypothesis. She merely makes the statement, conjectures as to why this result may have been found, and suggests that a different approach should be taken with this type of subject in future studies on upper-extremity weight bearing.

This brings us to the topic of what to do about the study that generates few data in support of the proposed hypotheses. Should this study be reported and published? Sometimes it is important that health professionals are given access to the results of such studies because:

- they may put to rest a popular myth that needs to be dispelled (see Box 10-H)
- or they may show that a particular methodology or research design is not a useful way to investigate a particular problem, thus saving others from making the same mistake
- or others may learn from the flaws and problems in the studies, which may then be redesigned to achieve the original purpose

In the final section of the paper, it is customary to remark on the shortcomings of the study, but it is not necessary to dwell on them. A simple acknowledgment is sufficient. Sometimes an instrument may have proved unreliable, subjects may have dropped out of the study, or there may have been some unforeseen interference with the study procedure. Whatever the problem, the reader will assume that you did what you could to correct for it and that you ran the study to the best of your ability. Giving readers the information will allow them to decide for themselves if the integrity of the study has been compromised (see Box 10-I).

Box 10-F

Van Deusen, Harlowe, and Baker (1989) report 1) similar findings to a study that used a wider age group than theirs and 2) inconsistent findings with a similar study in which the younger age group had been separated into two sections. The authors suggest that differences in findings in the latter case might have been due to the use of different measurement procedures. They also state that they cannot compare their project to yet a third study because the researchers had used different assessment tools.

Box 10–G

In Barnes's (1989) study on the relationship of upper-extremity weight bearing to hand skills of boys with cerebral palsy, the author states in the discussion:

The data on the left arm of Subject 4 are inconclusive. Subject 4's performance may have differed from that of Subject 5 and 6 because of his bilateral elbow contractures. The weightbearing treatment technique may not be as effective with subjects with contractures as with those free of joint limitations; therefore, alternate strategies for such patients should be considered.

(p. 241)

Box 10–H

Some writers have suggested that splinting would be helpful in increasing function for patients with hand contractures due to progressive systemic sclerosis. Seeger and Furst's study (1987) showed that this was not the case with their sample. Their abstract reads:

One of the major factors in the decreasing functional ability of patients with progressive systemic sclerosis is involvement of the patient's hands with secondary immobility and contractures. In a 2-month study of 19 patients, we assessed whether dynamic splinting could decrease proximal interphalangeal (PIP) flexion contractures. Of the eight patients who completed the study, one experienced a statistically significant improvement in PIP range of motion as a result of the splinting. There was no evidence that the use of splints served to maintain PIP extension when compared with the control hand.

(p. 118)

Box 10–I

While investigating the relationship between oral sensation and drooling in persons with cerebral palsy (Weiss-Lambrou, Tetreault, & Dudley, 1989), the researchers warn readers that their findings:

should be interpreted with caution because of the following methodological limitations: (a) the small sample size; (b) the poor test-retest reliability of the tests of oral stereognosis and oral form discrimination; and (c) the lack of data on interrater reliability.

The tests of oral sensation used in this study were not designed for persons with cerebral palsy; consequently, the major difficulty encountered in examining this parameter was the lack of oral sensation tests that are applicable with this population.

(p. 160)

Box 10–J

Davis and Bordieri (1988) not only suggest directions for further research based on their work, but also say why such research would be helpful to the profession:

. . . the next research step would be to identify strategies that foster perceived autonomy and that combat the disincentives reported by occupational therapists. This line of research would be invaluable to occupational therapy managers in today's competitive market who are seeking to attract, retain, and professionally motivate their staff members, and thus ensure the highest possible level of patient care.

(p. 595)

SUMMARY SECTION

Once you have interpreted your findings and drawn conclusions, it is usual to summarize what has happened during the study. In the summary, you are answering the questions 1) What have I contributed?, 2) How has my study helped to solve the original problem?, and 3) What conclusions and theoretical implications can I draw from my study? If the study is being written as an article for a professional journal, a paragraph is usually all that can be devoted to the summary due to space constraints. Trying to answer those three questions in a paragraph is a challenge, but can be done.

It is appropriate to briefly suggest improvements that could be made in the study procedures and design and to propose new research that may be appropriate based on your findings. These two items are especially important for the therapist interested in replicating or building upon your work (see Box 10–J).

Reporting the results of your study, interpreting them, and drawing conclusions are the last components of the research process. All that remains is getting the written report into suitable shape for publication (see Chapter 11).

STUMBLING BLOCKS

PICTORIAL DISPLAY OF DATA

Some professional journals have a limit on the number of pictorial representations (tables and figures) that may be used, because of reproduction costs. The Author's Guide, which is provided by the publisher, will probably mention any such limitation.

INTERPRETATIONS AND CONCLUSIONS

When interpreting your findings, the temptation is to try to make too much of the results. Investigators sometimes fall into the trap of extrapolating information and drawing conclusions that are not really warranted from the available data. It is important to stand back and critically review the data, asking yourself, "Am I justified in drawing this conclusion?" and "Is this really what the data mean?" Sometimes a colleague can offer an objective eye, should you become so embroiled in your own findings that you start drawing conclusions that are unwarranted.

WORKSHEETS

REPORTING RESULTS

Describe the sample in numerical terms:

Total number:

If subjects are people include:

Mean age:

Age range:

Number of males and females:

Qualifications:

Other attributes relevant to your study:

or

If subjects are records or other items, describe relevant characteristics:

Tabulate the data from your data sheets (these may be measurements from tests or equipment, returned surveys, recordings from interviews, data from client records, notations on observation sheets, etc.).

If you are using qualitative data:

Code your results, using the method you proposed earlier:

or

If you are using quantitative data:

Perform the statistical analyses on your tabulated data using the methods you proposed earlier. If you are working with a statistician, this is the time to take your material to him or her.

List your hypotheses here:

A.

B.

C.

D.

Review the results of the data analyses.

If you are using statistical techniques:

Did the findings reach significance levels for:

Hypothesis A. _____ Yes _____ No

B. _____ Yes _____ No

C. _____ Yes _____ No

D. _____ Yes _____ No

For each hypothesis that achieved significance, go back to the tabulated raw data to see the direction of the result (e.g., positive or negative, more of or less of, greater or smaller).

Go back and note beside each hypothesis whether or not it was supported by the data.

or

If you are using qualitative data:

Following your coding, does the preponderance of evidence suggest support for the hypotheses?

Hypothesis A. _____ Yes _____ No

B. _____ Yes _____ No

C. _____ Yes _____ No

D. _____ Yes _____ No

INTERPRETATIONS AND CONCLUSIONS

Turn to the literature review section and state if your findings agree with or depart from the findings of earlier studies you have mentioned.

Authors of study   Findings agree   Findings differ

For those findings that differ, speculate here as to what you think caused the difference.

Now, interpret your findings and draw conclusions for each hypothesis:

Hypothesis A

Hypothesis B

Hypothesis C

Hypothesis D

SUMMARY SECTION

Address the following questions:

What have I contributed here?

How has my study helped to solve the original problem?

What conclusions and theoretical implications can I draw from my study?

Mention any major shortcomings of the study:

Suggest improvements that could be made in the study design or procedures:

Propose new research that would build upon your study:

REFERENCES

Barnes, K. (1989). Direct replication: Relationship of upper extremity weight bearing to hand skills of boys with cerebral palsy. *Occupational Therapy Journal of Research, 9*(4), 235–242.

Davis, G., & Bordieri, J. (1988). Perceived autonomy and job satisfaction in occupational therapists. *American Journal of Occupational Therapy, 42*(9), 591–595.

Revak, J. (1989). Incidence of upper extremity discomfort among piano students. *American Journal of Occupational Therapy, 43*(3), 149–154.

Schwartzberg, S. L. (1982). Motivation for activities of daily living: A study of selected psychiatric patients' self-reports. *Occupational Therapy in Mental Health, 2*(3), 1–26.

Seeger, M. W., & Furst, D. E. (1987). Effects of splinting in the treatment of hand contractures in progressive systemic sclerosis. *American Journal of Occupational Therapy, 41*(2), 118–121.

Steinbeck, T. M. (1986). Purposeful activity and performance. *American Journal of Occupational Therapy, 40*(8), 529–534.

Van Deusen, J., Harlowe, D., & Baker, L. (1989). Body image perceptions of the community-based elderly. *Occupational Therapy Journal of Research, 9*(4), 243–248.

Weiss-Lambrou, R., Tetreault, S., & Dudley, J. (1989). The relationship between oral sensation and drooling in persons with cerebral palsy. *American Journal of Occupational Therapy, 43*(3), 155–161.

Additional Reading

Cox, R., & West, W. (1986). Chapter 7: Dealing with data. In *Fundamentals of research for health professionals* (pp. 67–87). Laurel, MD: RAMSCO Publishing Co.

Currier, D. P. (1984). Chapter 12: Revealing research. In *Elements of research in physical therapy* (pp. 297–323). Baltimore: Williams & Wilkins.

Ethridge, D., & McSweeney, M. (1971). Research in occupational therapy: 5. Data interpretation, results and conclusions. *American Journal of Occupational Therapy, XXV*(3), 149–154.

Gonnella, C. (1973). Let's reduce the understanding gap: 4. Data presentation: Guidelines for authors (and readers). *Physical Therapy, 53*, 871–875.

Morris, B., Fitz-Gibbon, J., & Freeman C. (1987). *How to communicate research findings.* Newbury Park, CA: Sage Publications.

Oyster, C. K., Hanten, W. P., & Llorens, L. A. (1987). Chapter 15: Communicating research. In *Introduction to research: A guide for the health science professional* (pp. 190–207). Philadelphia: J.B. Lippincott.

11

Writing and Publishing

You have made it through to the final stage, but don't sit back and think you have finished! No research project is complete until the results are shared. Unfortunately, this is often the point at which investigators run out of steam, and the material languishes in a drawer waiting to be written. Until colleagues are informed about the findings of the study, those findings are not useful. The only benefit up to this point is that you have had the opportunity to conduct a piece of research.

If you have completed the worksheets in this book as you went along, you will have done most of the work involved in writing the study. When carrying out future research projects, if you can bring yourself to do the writing as you conduct each phase of a project, producing the final written product will be far less formidable. This does not mean that the material is written in its final form but rather that the thinking and planning you went through are captured on paper. It is then a relatively simple matter to put those notes into a suitable form, either for publication in a journal or as a thesis. The format and amount of detail for journal publications and for theses are quite different, and the two will be addressed separately. Journal publication will be addressed first.

PUBLISHING IN A JOURNAL

If you wish to submit your work for publication in a professional journal, you will need to select an appropriate publication, find out about the required writing style, write up your work in that format, submit the article, wait for the review process, make requested revisions, and comply with copyright procedures.

CHOOSING A JOURNAL

You may already have decided upon the professional journal to which you will be submitting your study. Sometimes it is clear that one is more appropriate than another. For occupational therapists and physical therapists, the choices are usually the *American Journal of Occupational Therapy*, *Physical Therapy*, the *Occupational Therapy Journal of Research*, *Occupational Therapy in Mental Health*, *Physical and Occupational Therapy Journal in Pediatrics*, or *Physical and Occupational Therapy Journal in Geriatrics*. Other publications you might consider include *Physiotherapy Canada*, the *Canadian Journal of Occupational Therapy*, the *British Journal of Physiotherapy*, or the *British Journal of*

Occupational Therapy. Other health- and sociology-related journals are included in Appendix K in the back of this book.

Look in back issues of the journals you are considering for the aim and scope of the publication (often in the first issue of each year), so that you can see which organization is responsible for publishing the journal, the aim and purpose of the journal, the professional fields addressed by the journal, topics that are generally published in the journal, features of the journal besides articles, and the type of review process to which articles are subjected. This information may influence your decision to submit your work to that particular journal. Sometimes the aim and scope of a publication are printed on the back page of the journal, often in the January or December issue. The circulation may be mentioned somewhere in the journal so that you can see how many of your colleagues the publication will reach.

While you are looking for the journal's aim and scope, you should look also for the Author's Guide or Information for Authors. Author's Guides are often printed at the end of the journal annually or more frequently. This will give information about the writing style used by the journal, how many manuscript pages are acceptable, and any specific requirements the publication may have regarding photographs, drawings, figures, and so forth. A sample of Instructions to Authors from *Physical Therapy* and the Author's Guide for the *American Journal of Occupational Therapy* is given in Appendix M.

Always look through several copies of any journal you are considering to be sure it is the kind of publication in which you would like your article to appear. It may be helpful to browse in the journal room of a well-stocked library to get an idea of appropriate publications. Most libraries display the current month's journals in alphabetical order by title, so you can quickly pick out titles that appear appropriate. The following publications also may be of assistance to prospective authors: *Author's Guide to Journals in the Health Field* (Ardell & James, 1980), *Author's Guide to Journals in Psychology, Psychiatry, and Social Work* (Markle & Rinn, 1977), and *Author's Guide to Journals in Sociology and Related Fields* (Sussman, 1978). These three books are available in the reference section of most libraries and provide the name of the journal, the publishing organization, frequency of publication, circulation, professional fields addressed, major topics covered, percentage of articles accepted, and the review process. *Magazines for Libraries* (Katz & Sternberg Katz, 1986) lists periodicals alphabetically, by title, and under subject areas given in the table of contents. The frequency of publication, price, circulation, suitable audience, publisher, and whether articles are peer reviewed are listed for each periodical. The table of contents includes these topics: Disabilities, Rehabilitation, Medicine and Health, Aging, Psychology, Sports Medicine, Sociology, and Occupational Health. The publishers are dependent upon editors to update the information in all four publications; consequently the data are sometimes not current.

Most editors request that you do not submit your manuscript to any other journal while it is under consideration by them. Once your article has been accepted for publication, you may be required to sign a copyright form.

WRITING STYLES

After you have selected a journal, you need to find out which writing style is used. There are several styles in use, but many health-related journals subscribe to the style described in the *Publication Manual of the American Psychological Association* APA, 1983. The *American Journal of Occupational Therapy*, the *Occupational Therapy Journal of Research, Occupational Therapy in Mental Health*, and *Physical Therapy and Occupational Therapy in Geriatrics* all use this style manual, while *Physical Therapy* uses the American Physical Therapy Association (APTA) *Style Manual* (1987). *Physical Therapy and Occupational Therapy in Pediatrics*, on the other hand, requires the Index Medicus style as outlined by the *Stylebook/Editorial Manual* (1971) of the American Medical Association. Most journals will accept an article for review only if it is written in the required style.

The format for writing a research article is detailed in the APA and APTA publication manuals; you should use these manuals during the writing process. Most libraries will have the manuals, but it is highly recommended that you obtain your own copy. The manuals give useful information about such general topics as the quality of content; types of articles; length, headings, and tone; parts of a manuscript; and guidelines for specific items such as non-sexist language, punctuation, abbreviations, quotations, tables and figures, references and reference lists, footnotes, and typing.

FORMAT FOR A JOURNAL ARTICLE

The general format for a scientific journal article tends to be similar in most journals. Customary sections are Problem, Background, Purpose, Hypotheses, Method, Results, and Discussion. Each section is described below. All of the material to be included in your paper can be obtained from the worksheets you have completed. You are now ready to start writing your article in its final form.

Problem

Present the problem that you described in the Problem Statement worksheet following Chapter 3. This is the major issue you wished to address by conducting your study. Tell readers why this is an important problem and one that needs a solution. Are there clients who will benefit or programs that will be improved? Using the material you wrote in the Background section following Chapter 3, answer for readers the question "What is wrong in society or a patient's life that this study will help?"

Next, summarize in a sentence or two how the hypotheses and experimental design relate to the problem. In other words, how will your particular study address the larger problem. Finally, mention the theoretical implications of the study—what is likely to be improved as a result of your study.

This whole section should not be more than a paragraph or two and should give the reader a firm sense of what was done and why.

Background

Most of the Background section of an article will come from the literature review you conducted. Discuss the literature but do not include an exhaustive historical review. This is the section that will be most condensed, given all the material you have amassed. Most journals have space constraints such that they will not accept more than one or two paragraphs concerning the background literature. However, a publication such as the *Occupational Therapy Journal of Research* may allow more space because the journal specializes in research papers and a considerable amount of space is allowed for each article. The APA Manual provides useful guidelines for writing the Background section (see Box 11–A). Point out the logical continuity between previous work and your work on the topic. Controversial issues should be treated fairly, and studies supporting both sides of the argument should be presented.

Box 11–A

"Although you should acknowledge the contributions of others to the study of the problem, cite only that research pertinent to the specific issue and avoid references with only tangential or general significance. If you summarize earlier works, avoid nonessential details: instead, emphasize pertinent findings, relevant methodological issues, and major conclusions. Refer the reader to general surveys or reviews of the topic if they are available."
(American Psychological Association, 1983, p. 25)

Purpose

Now that you have introduced the problem and given readers the background to the problem, you should state your purpose in carrying out the study. Tell readers what you hoped to accomplish and why your study, above all others, was worth doing. You have already written these statements in the Purpose and Significance sections of the worksheets following Chapter 3.

Hypotheses

In this section, you simply state the hypotheses or null hypotheses or research questions. A formal statement will give clarity to the paper.

Method

This section describes in detail how the study was conducted. It should contain sufficient detail to allow other researchers to replicate the study and for readers to assess both the appropriateness of your methods to the purpose of the study and the reliability and validity of the study. The Method section of the article should contain the material you described following Chapters 4, 5, and 6 and may be divided into subsections covering *subjects*, *materials/instruments*, and *procedures*. You have already written information on these three items in the protocol at the end of Chapter 5.

Subjects

Subjects are data sources for research studies and are the people or items from which you have gathered data. In writing the subject section, you should describe the criteria used to determine the population for the study, stating which literature indicates that these criteria are necessary or desirable. Then, the method of sample selection should be described (i.e., random or non-random selection). If non-random selection was used, was a convenience sample used or some other method? The method of assigning subjects to groups should be addressed, if relevant. Add how many subjects were in the study and how many were included in each group. If there was any subject attrition during the study, this also should be mentioned.

Instruments

All the data collection methods used should be listed in this section. The information can be obtained from the worksheets following Chapter 7. You need to include any information you found on reliability and validity. If the measure was devised by you specifically for the study, this should be mentioned. In this case, it may be useful to include a copy of the instrument in the article. There should be a complete description of how the data collection methods were administered, including whether a pre-test and post-test were used, who administered the test, whether the test was administered in a group or individually, the environmental conditions, and how long the data collection took.

Procedures

This section should spell out each step undertaken during the study. The information can be found in the Research Protocol you wrote and in the Method section of the Proposal for the Human Subjects Committee. Ideally, this section should be written in sufficient detail that the study could be replicated; however, journal space constraints often negate this possibility. In most professional journals, the author's name and address are printed with the article so that interested readers can write and request further information.

Results

In the Results section, briefly summarize the main findings, then report the data in detail so that you may justify the conclusions that will be drawn later. Discussing implications is not appropriate in the Results section; just stick to the facts. Remember to use pictorial representations for large sets of data such as tables, graphs, and charts.

When reporting the findings from inferential statistics such as t tests, chi-squares, or f tests, include information on the significance level and the degrees of freedom. The style manuals give information on how to type statistical results, for example, when to use small and large letters such as n for sample and N for population and when to underline such as in t test.

Discussion

Here is your chance to enjoy yourself and speculate on what the results mean. At first writing, jot down all the ideas that come to mind about your findings; then in later drafts, you can expand on meaningful theories and discard those that are not useful or valid. Don't be afraid to interpret your findings, but remember that you can discuss an issue only if you mentioned its findings in the Results section. Material for this final section will come from the worksheets following Chapter 10.

The opening statement of the discussion should inform the reader whether or not the hypothesis was supported or the research question was answered. Then you are free to draw upon the literature, discussing similarities and differences in the findings of your study and the studies mentioned in the literature review. You must state findings that do not support your hypotheses and briefly speculate on why they might have come about and what they might mean.

At one time, it was customary to end with a paragraph reviewing the study and its main findings, but this is less necessary now because most journals are printing an abstract at the beginning of the article.

References

The reference list and referencing in the text are the most common places to make typographical errors and errors in style. Using APA format (which has been used throughout this book), you should use the authors' last names and year of publication in the text (or solely the year if the names already appear in the text). In the reference list, you should give authors' last name, initials, year in parentheses, title of article or book (underline title of book), publisher of book or name of journal (name of journal underlined), volume number (underlined), issue number, and page numbers of article. Using APTA style, references in the text are indicated by superscripts following the name and are numbered consecutively throughout the text. They are typed consecutively in a separate reference list at the end of the completed text. In the reference list, you should give authors' last name, initials, title of article or book, name of journal or publisher of book, page numbers, and year of publication. Samples are given in Box 11–B.

It is a good idea to have a colleague go through the entire manuscript with you, one reading the references in the text and the other checking the reference list, to ensure that names and dates match. Journal editors hold authors responsible for the accuracy of references.

Box 11–B

Sample citation and reference from *Physical Therapy:*

Auricular TENS significantly decreased pain in fifteen patients suffering with various distal extremity disorders.[11]

11. Longobardi AG, Clelland JA, Knowles CJ, et al: Effects of auricular transcutaneous electrical nerve stimulation on distal extremity pain: A pain study. Phys Ther 69:10–17, 1989

Sample citation and reference from the *American Journal of Occupational Therapy:*

A major goal of occupational therapy is to enhance a person's ability to interact in the environment in a competent manner (Rogers, 1982).

Rogers, J. C. (1982). Guest Editorial—Educating the inquisitive practitioner. *Occupational Therapy Journal of Research, 2*, 3–11.

Abstract

Most journals require an abstract of the article and specify a number of words the abstract may not exceed; for example, the *American Journal of Occupational Therapy* has a maximum abstract length of 150 words. In summarizing your article, the content should be factual; that is, state only events that occurred, items that were used, or data that were found, rather than opinions or suppositions. While being succinct by necessity and definition, an abstract also should be "sufficiently complete to enable the reader to grasp the essence of the paper quickly" (AJOT, 1990, p. 92). Typically an abstract will contain a statement of the problem, method of study, results, and conclusions. Boxes 11–C and 11–D give abstracts from the *American Journal of Occupational Therapy* and *Physical Therapy*.

MAKING IT INTERESTING

Scientific writing may be different from literary writing, but that does not mean that is has to be boring. Although reporting on research in an interesting manner is a challenge, it can be done. The writing should not lack style or be dull. Present your research and your findings directly, but aim for an interesting and compelling style that shows readers how involved you are with the project. Your involvement should be infectious and make readers want to read on to see what happens. The APA Manual offers useful advice on the expression of ideas (see Box 11–E).

The manual gives excellent suggestions for the orderly presentation of ideas, smoothness of expression, economy of expression, precision and clarity in word choice, strategies to improve writing style, and grammar (pp. 32–36). Reading this section may prove inspiring to the would-be author of an article.

Box 11–C

"In this pilot study, we investigated the clinical use of the Miller Assessment for Preschoolers (MAP) (Miller, 1982) with a sample of children with suspected or confirmed developmental delays. A retrospective chart audit was performed for 95 subjects, 30 girls and 65 boys, 34 to 68 months of age. Clinically related diagnoses were classified into six medical/developmental groups and a no-diagnosis group, some of the MAP score patterns differed significantly (p < .01). These score patterns provide preliminary evidence for the MAP's effectiveness in screening children with developmental delays."
(Daniels & Bressler, 1990, p. 48)

Box 11–D

"The study was designed to provide a quantitative analysis of toe-walking in children with cerebral palsy (CP). The total internal moment developed about the ankle joint during locomotion and the passive component of this internal moment were measured. The contributions of the active and passive components were expressed as the ratio (R) between the passive moment and the total internal moment. Measurements were compared for 13 children with CP and 5 healthy children. For the data analysis, the children with CP exhibiting apparently similar toe-walking, were divided into 2 groups: 1) Group CPI and 2) Group CPII. Group CPI was characterized by a small ratio R value, which indicated the presence of excessive contractions of the triceps surae muscle during locomotion. In Group CPII, the ratio R value was abnormally high, which indicated that a contracture (ie, structural change of the muscle or the tendon) was entirely or at least partly responsible for toe-walking. Each group requires a different therapeutic strategy."

(Tardieu, Lespargot, Tabary, & Bret, 1989, p. 656)

PROCEDURES FOR PUBLICATION

Once you have selected the journal of your choice and prepared your article according to the appropriate format, you are ready to mail in your work. Be sure to follow the directions for number of copies, typing style, page numbering, spacing, and so on. Include a cover letter stating the name of the article together with any covering statements you were asked to make in the Author's Guide. These often include a statement to the effect that your paper is not under consideration by any other publication and that you will be willing to sign a copyright form.

Sometimes you will receive a card from the editor saying that the article has been received and that the review process has begun. Now be prepared for a long wait — several months. At this point, the editor will send copies of your article to three or four reviewers, usually experts in your field and in the area of specialization of the study. Often reviewers are asked to answer a series of questions that will help the editor decide 1) if the topic is relevant to the readership, 2) if it has been appropriately covered, 3) if it is timely, and 4) if the study was reasonable and of good quality. Once all the reviews are returned, the editor will make a decision whether to accept the article as it is, to accept it with revisions, or to reject the article. As you can imagine, it takes several months for you to receive the letter containing this decision.

If you hear from the editor that your article has been rejected for publication, you will usually be told the reason for rejection. Perhaps the topic is unsuitable for the readership or is considered untimely, or reviewers do not consider the project of a standard worthy for publication. Do not be discouraged. Submit your work to another journal, perhaps spending more time matching your content to that of the journal.

Often editors will accept an article, providing the author agrees to make some changes. It can be discouraging to see one's work returned covered with red pencil markings, but the requested changes are often not as major as they may at first appear. Occasionally, revisions are requested that would not improve the article or that would alter the author's

---

Box 11–E

"Clear communication, which is the prime objective of scientific writing, may be achieved by presenting ideas in an orderly manner and by expressing oneself smoothly and precisely. By developing ideas clearly and logically, you invite readers to read, encourage them to continue, and make their task agreeable by leading them smoothly from thought to thought."

(American Psychological Association, 1983, p. 31)

meaning or intent. It is not necessary to make these changes. Merely explain why they would not be beneficial, and perhaps suggest a rewrite that would clarify your meaning. Make reasonable alterations quickly and send back the revised copy within a couple of weeks.

Do not be surprised if your article goes back and forth between you and the editor a few more times before it is acceptable. Above all, do not become discouraged so that you stop revising and resubmitting. If the editor considers the material suitable for publication, it is merely a question of time before you have it in publishable form.

When your article is finally ready, the editor may ask you to sign a copyright form stating that you hand over the publishing rights of your article to that publication. You also will be informed that your article is being sent to the printer to be prepared for publication and that you will shortly receive page proofs. You must read the proofs immediately to check for errors and mail them back. The time frame is extremely tight because publications are scheduled for release immediately after they are printed. Sometimes you will be asked to telephone in any changes in the page proofs to speed up the process. Only minor changes, such as spelling or punctuation corrections, can be made in proofs. It is too late to rewrite sentences or make any major changes in context.

After that, nothing remains to be done except to sit back and wait to see your name in print. Some publications will send you a complementary copy of the journal in which your article appears, while others will send you several copies of the article alone. Now you really have finished. You have something to show for all your effort, something you can be proud of, and you have made a contribution to your profession. It was worth it, wasn't it?

THESIS PREPARATION

Preparing a thesis requires a somewhat different series of steps and considerations. The procedural steps involved usually consist of:

1. Preparing a thesis proposal and presenting it to your chosen thesis committee at a thesis proposal hearing; making required changes.
2. Preparing materials for a human subjects committee review; presenting or submitting materials to the human subjects committee responsible for your facility; making required changes; presenting or submitting materials to the human subjects committee of the facility in which the research will be performed (if relevant); making required changes.
3. Implementing the research project.
4. Preparing the written thesis and defending it before your thesis committee at a thesis defense meeting; making required changes; preparing the thesis document for binding and presentation to the required sites, such as your department or college library.

Although these are customary procedures involved in the preparation of a thesis, they may be different at your institution. You should follow the procedures used there.

WRITING STYLE

As with journal articles, required writing styles will vary from college to college. In occupational therapy and physical therapy programs, the style used is often that of the American Psychological Association or the American Physical Therapy Association, but you should check with your department to be sure. Again, it is advisable to obtain a copy of the relevant style manual, because you will probably need to refer to it frequently during the writing process.

THESIS PROPOSAL FORMAT

There may be a required format for a thesis proposal in use at your college. If so, it will probably be similar to the following format.

The front page should show the title of the study, the name of the researcher, the date of the proposal, and the names of the thesis readers.

Description and Rationale for the Study

Introduction

You may choose to have an introduction or you may move right into the Problem Statement. If you have an introduction, it should be brief and set the stage for the problem to be investigated.

Problem statement

This material may be found on the Problem Statement worksheets following Chapter 3 and should state clearly the problem your study will address.

Background

Here you will state the need for the study: why the problem is of pressing concern. The material comes from the literature review you conducted and generally will not exceed two or three pages. It should include several people's opinion regarding the problem's importance and the need for study, together with some general facts about the nature, extent, and seriousness of the problem.

Purpose

State what you wish to do about the problem by carrying out your study. Gather the material from the Purpose section of the worksheets following Chapter 3.

Significance

This is the "so what?" of your study. What will be changed as a result of your study? Use the material on the worksheets following Chapter 3.

Literature review

At this stage of thesis preparation, you will probably have conducted only a preliminary literature review, so this section should contain a list of the topics your in-depth review will cover. However, you should try to include one or two studies that support your view that the problem is important as well as some studies using similar and dissimilar research methods to the method you propose to use for investigating the problem.

Design of the Study

Research question or hypotheses

Here you simply state the research question(s), or hypotheses or null hypotheses. A formal statement will give clarity to the proposal.

Assumptions

List the assumptions you are making in designing the study, using the material on the Assumptions worksheet following Chapter 6.

Scope and limitations

Describe the scope of your study and outline the limitations that are apparent so far. This material can be found on the worksheets following Chapter 6.

Research design

This should be a simple statement of your decision about the research design you will use and is the decision you made after you read Chapter 5.

Research method

Subjects: Include the criteria you will use to define the population, the method you will use to select the sample, how many will be in the sample, and the method you will use to assign the subjects to experimental and control groups. All of this material will be found in the Subject worksheet following Chapter 6.

Variables: Define the dependent and independent variables if you are doing experimental or quasi-experimental research; define the variables being correlated if you are doing correlational research.

Definition of terms: List the terms that will have a simple definition; then operationalize those terms that will play an important role in your study—usually those mentioned in the hypotheses. You did this task when you completed the worksheets following Chapter 6.

Procedures: This section comprises the step-by-step account of your research project as you listed it in the protocol you wrote at the end of Chapter 5. Included here are the procedures to be used to ensure subject confidentiality, to obtain subjects' informed consent, and to ensure that necessary treatment will not be withheld, as well as statements concerning the risk/benefit ratio to subjects and the safety of the study. You prepared this material for inclusion in the packet of material for the human subjects committee on worksheets following Chapter 9.

Data collection instruments: List all the methods you will be using to collect data from the subjects. Describe the methods/tests/measures, give reliability and validity (if available), state when in the research process the administration will occur. This material may be found on the worksheets following Chapter 7.

Data analysis: This is the method you propose to use to analyze the data you will collect. It is possible that your methods may change, once you have actually gone through the experience of data gathering, but thesis committee members will want to see that you have thought about the analyses and that you have an idea of the procedures you will use. You have thought this process through on the worksheets following Chapter 7 if you are gathering qualitative data and Chapter 8 if you are gathering quantitative data.

Timetable

Some departments require thesis writers to plan a timetable for the process of thesis preparation. This forces the student to think about how much time each step will take and encourages realistic planning for the entire process. In plotting a timetable, you should include actual dates by which events will happen, rather than merely stating that a literature review will take 3 months, for example. In the Preface of this book, some information was given about estimating time frames for conducting research and some sample timetables are shown in Appendix N.

Resources

Sometimes students are asked to list the resources they anticipate needing to complete their thesis. If you are asked to do so, you should consider whether you will need assistance with typing, editing, or proofreading; the help of a statistician; the use of a computer for statistical computation or for word processing; access to library facilities; access to patients or clients who meet your selection criteria; the use of treatment equipment or materials; or assistance from other therapists in carrying out the treatment or in testing subjects.

Reference list

The reference list for a proposal should be complete and written in the style that will be required for the completed thesis. You should find out what that style will be, acquire the appropriate style manual, and study the section on referencing.

Appendices

The appendices usually included in a thesis proposal are tests, measures, or data-gathering instruments; forms to gather subjects' informed consent to participate in the study; and other forms that may be required by the human subjects committee that are specific to the study.

PROCEDURES FOR THE PROPOSAL

You will have been working with your thesis committee members, often known as thesis readers, in the preparation of the proposal. The completed proposal should be submitted to each committee member at least a week before the scheduled hearing date so that they have time to review it. You should bring your own copy of the proposal to the hearing and be prepared to answer questions about the underlying philosophy and theory, the design and methodology, or the importance and relevance of your proposed study. This is, after all, what you propose to do to meet the department's requirements for a thesis, and your readers will expect that you have thought through the project carefully and that you are able to discuss it knowledgeably.

There will undoubtedly be discussions about certain portions of the proposal, with exchange of ideas about alterations and improvements. There should be no surprises if you have worked with readers ahead of time in the preparation of the proposal; nevertheless, some readers are inspired when involved in discussions with colleagues and at the hearing may well make good suggestions for improvements. Unless you feel strongly that the suggestions would not improve the study, you should make the required changes, resubmit the proposal, and get the go-ahead to start your research.

Before you can actually start, however, you need to prepare and present materials to the human subjects committee. This procedure was described in Chapter 9 and, if you completed the worksheets, you will have most of the material in place. Some of it may need revising following your proposal hearing. Assuming that the human subjects committee approved your study and all else went well, you may now carry out the study.

THESIS FORMAT

The final step is to write the material in thesis form. It is possible that your college has an idiosyncratic format for thesis writing, but in all probability, the form will be similar to that found in Figure 11–1. The basis for the information needed for the thesis can be found on the worksheets you completed at the end of each chapter of this book. The relevant chapter is listed following each topic heading in Figure 11–1. You have probably written a bare-bones statement or two for each component and now need to fill in the details.

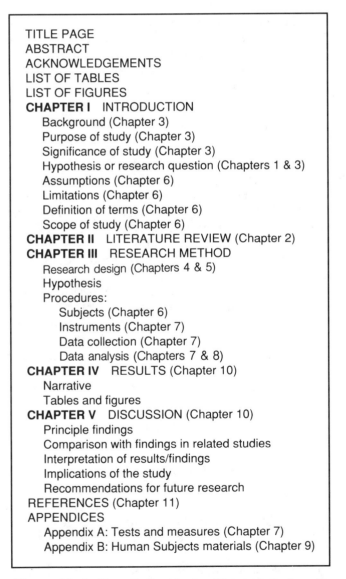

```
TITLE PAGE
ABSTRACT
ACKNOWLEDGEMENTS
LIST OF TABLES
LIST OF FIGURES
CHAPTER I   INTRODUCTION
    Background (Chapter 3)
    Purpose of study (Chapter 3)
    Significance of study (Chapter 3)
    Hypothesis or research question (Chapters 1 & 3)
    Assumptions (Chapter 6)
    Limitations (Chapter 6)
    Definition of terms (Chapter 6)
    Scope of study (Chapter 6)
CHAPTER II   LITERATURE REVIEW (Chapter 2)
CHAPTER III   RESEARCH METHOD
    Research design (Chapters 4 & 5)
    Hypothesis
    Procedures:
        Subjects (Chapter 6)
        Instruments (Chapter 7)
        Data collection (Chapter 7)
        Data analysis (Chapters 7 & 8)
CHAPTER IV   RESULTS (Chapter 10)
    Narrative
    Tables and figures
CHAPTER V   DISCUSSION (Chapter 10)
    Principle findings
    Comparison with findings in related studies
    Interpretation of results/findings
    Implications of the study
    Recommendations for future research
REFERENCES (Chapter 11)
APPENDICES
    Appendix A: Tests and measures (Chapter 7)
    Appendix B: Human Subjects materials (Chapter 9)
```

Figure 11–1 Format for thesis. Chapter numbers in parentheses indicate where information for each section is located in this book.

PROCEDURES FOR THE THESIS

Most readers prefer to read one or two thesis chapters at a time, as they are written. This way they can be sure the student is on track, and necessary changes may be made as the writing progresses. If a reader does not ask you for chapters as you write, it is a good idea to request this type of review to be sure that you are using the correct style before getting too far along in the process. Even so, when your readers see the entire manuscript, they will undoubtedly have suggestions for change and will probably want some sections rewritten.

As soon as all the readers are satisfied with the content, a thesis defense should be scheduled. This is a meeting during which you will "defend" your thesis. The defense is often an open meeting, which others may attend. It usually takes the form of a question-and-answer period followed by a general discussion about your project, but ask your first reader about the format of the meetings at your college so that you can be prepared.

The outcome of a defense meeting is usually that the thesis is approved as is or it is approved as long as minor changes are made. If a student is asked to make major revisions, this is usually an indication that the student did not work closely enough with committee members during the actual writing.

When all the readers are satisfied with the final product, and the approval sheets have been signed indicating that the student has completed the requirements for the thesis, all that remains is to make the required number of copies and deliver them to the appropriate sites. Colleges usually require copies of theses for the department and/or college libraries; also professional association libraries may request a copy.

PREPARING THE THESIS FOR PUBLICATION

Sometimes, students are interested in preparing their thesis for publication. This is an excellent idea and probably should happen more often than it does; however, it is not a simple job because so much cutting and rewriting is necessary. It is difficult to bring oneself to eliminate so much hard-won material! One of the readers might be willing to help and may be more objective about which portions can be ruthlessly discarded, while retaining the sense of the work. Generally, the literature review is the chapter that is most massacred. In fact, it must be boiled down to about two to four paragraphs for most journals—quite a daunting feat from 15 or 20 pages.

If you plan to rework your thesis for publication, the best plan might be to return to the worksheets you prepared during the project and to make a fresh start directly from the worksheets. Sometimes it is simpler to write something from scratch than to rework material that is written for another purpose. If this sounds like a good idea to you, you should refer to the first half of this chapter and follow the sequence of writing for publishing in a journal.

STUMBLING BLOCKS

The point at which many studies get bogged down rather than being published is when the author receives the article from the editor and sees that yet more work is needed to get it into publishable shape. Many first-time authors think that drafting the article the first time is all there is to it and that it will be acceptable that way. Most of us quickly learn that this is not so. What appears to us to be a flawless piece of work may appear to others as a piece that can be improved.

Generally, the revisions are not as major as they might first appear. As soon as you have recovered from the first disappointment, go through the recommendations one by one to get a more realistic feeling for items that can be changed quickly and sections that will require more work. You may be surprised at how simple some of the revisions are to make.

As the author, you may be too close to the topic to see alternative ways of presenting ideas. A colleague may help shed a more objective light on things and might have suggestions for the more major revisions.

What can be even more discouraging is that some of the requests for changes may, in the author's view, change the meaning of the writing or may not represent what the author wanted to say. You are under no obligation to make these changes. In such a case, you should write to the editor explaining your concern and stating that you do not feel that altering the text, on that particular point, would be beneficial. Editors are reasonable people and by and large will agree with you. If they do not, however, you should decide how important the point is to you. If it is very important, you may choose to withdraw your article from that particular publication and submit it to another. Always let an editor know if this is what you are doing.

I would recommend that you set a deadline by which you will make all the changes—perhaps within 2 weeks. In my experience, if you do not get past this stage quickly, the "rejected" manuscript will sit in a drawer permanently. As mentioned earlier, this is the point at which many first-time authors' manuscripts languish and die.

WORKSHEETS

If you are preparing your study for publication in a professional journal:

CHOOSING THE BEST JOURNAL FOR YOUR STUDY

You must decide on the journal of your choice. If this is not immediately clear to you, visit a library and review the journals on display in the journal room. If none of the journals on display looks exactly right, look through the Author's Guide to Journals series.

List possible journals here:

Appropriate

A. _____ ___Yes ___No
B. _____ ___Yes ___No
C. _____ ___Yes ___No
D. _____ ___Yes ___No
E. _____ ___Yes ___No

Review the aim and scope, and check off if the journals still seem appropriate.

Pick three of the most promising journals and look through several recent copies of each to see if your study fits the journals' style and content.

Make your first choice of journal:

WRITING STYLE

Review the Author's Guide to find which writing style is used. State here:

Obtain a copy of this writing style guide.

Review the guide before you start writing.

WRITING

Gather your worksheets from previous chapters and arrange them in sections:

Problem
Background
Purpose
Hypothesis
Method
Results
Discussion

Following the information in this chapter, embellish the material on the **Problem** worksheet, getting it into its final form:

Statement of **Purpose**:

Now write the **Background** section, working from your Literature Review worksheets:

Write out your **Hypotheses:**

Describe the **Method**, including:

Subjects:

Instruments:

Procedures:

Give the **Results**:

Now, discuss your **Conclusions**:

Was the hypothesis supported?

Make comparisons with the literature findings:

Your interpretations and conclusions:

Any limitations:

Suggestions for future research:

Compose the reference list:

Write an abstract:

Go back and review your work.

It is interesting?

Does it tell what was done and what happened—clearly and succinctly?

Are your interpretations and conclusions justified?

PROCEDURES FOR PUBLICATION

Review the Author's Guide again to be sure you have followed all the instructions.

Print the required number of copies of your article.

Write a cover letter to the editor.

Mail the package to the editor by first class mail.

REFERENCES

American Journal of Occupational Therapy. (1990). Author's Guide. *American Journal of Occupational Therapy, 44*(1), 92–93.

American Medical Association. (1971). *Stylebook/editorial manual.* New York: Author.

American Physical Therapy Association. (1987). *Style manual* (5th ed.) Alexandria, VA: Author.

American Psychological Association. (1983). *Publication manual of the American Psychological Association* (3rd ed.) Washington, DC: Author.

Ardell, D., & James, J. (Eds.). (1980). *Author's guide to journals in the health field,* New York: Haworth Press.

Daniels, L. E., & Bressler, S. (1990). The Miller Assessment for Preschoolers: Clinical use with children with developmental delays. *American Journal of Occupational Therapy, 44*(1), 48–53.

Katz, B., & Sternberg Katz, L. (Eds.) (1986). *Magazines for Libraries.* NY: R.R. Bowker.

Liu, H. I., Currier, D. P., & Threlkeld, A. J. (1987). Circulatory response of digital arteries associated with electrical stimulation of calf muscle in healthy subjects. *Physical Therapy, 67*(3), 340–345.

Markle, A., & Rinn, R. C. (Eds.). (1977). *Author's guide to journals in psychology, psychiatry and social work.* New York: Haworth Press.

Sussman, M. B. (Ed.). (1978). *Author's guide to journals in sociology and related fields.* New York: Haworth Press.

Tardieu, C., Lespargot, A., Tabary, C., & Bret, M. (1989). Toe-walking in children with cerebral palsy: Contributions of contracture and excessive contraction of triceps surae muscle. *Physical Therapy, 69*(8), 656–662.

ADDITIONAL READING

Bates, J. D. (1980). *Writing with precision: How to write so that you cannot possibly be misunderstood.* Washington, DC: Acropolis Books.

Carter, J., & Sylvester, P. (1987). *Writing for your peers: The primary journal paper.* New York: Praeger.

Copperud, R. H. (1980). *American usage and style: The consensus.* New York: Van Nostrand Reinhold.

Day, R. A. (1979). *How to write and publish a scientific paper.* Philadelphia: ISI Press.

Ethridge, D. A., & McSweeney, M. (1971). Research in occupational therapy: 6. Research writing. *American Journal of Occupational Therapy, XXV*(4), 210–214.

International Association of Business Communicators. (1982). *Without bias: A guidebook for nondiscriminatory communication.* New York: John Wiley & Sons.*

Ross-Larson, B. (1982). *Edit yourself.* New York: Norton.

Skillin, M. E., & Gay, R. M. (1974). *Words into type.* Englewood Cliffs, NJ: Prentice-Hall.

Strunk, W., Jr., & White, E. B. (1979). *The elements of style* (3rd ed.). New York: Macmillan.

*Provides guidelines for language that is free of bias of ethnicity, sex, age, and disability.

APPENDIX

Indexes and Abstracts

Abstracts for Social Workers. Quarterly. Abstracts from journals of social work under: social policy and action, service methods, fields of service, the social work profession, history of social work, related fields in the social sciences.

Abstracts of Hospital Management Studies. Quarterly. International abstracts of studies on management, planning, and public policy related to health care delivery.

Ageline. Produced by American Association for Retired Persons. More than 16,500 documents on all aspects of gerontology. Bimonthly updates.

Biological Abstracts. Semimonthly. International abstracts of periodicals including behavioral sciences, bioinstrumentation, environmental biology, genetics, nutrition, and public health.

Child Development Abstracts. Three times per year. Abstracts of articles and books in a wide variety of fields as they relate to infancy and child development.

Combined Health Information Database. Produced by National Institutes of Health. More than 24,000 documents combining four health-related data bases: arthritis, diabetes, health education, digestive diseases. Quarterly updates.

Compendex. Produced by Engineering Information Inc. More than 1,102,100 documents on all aspects of engineering and technology including rehabilitation engineering. Monthly updates.

Cumulative Index to Nursing and Allied Health Literature. From 1956 to present. Indexes all major nursing journals, plus book reviews, pamphlets, films, and recordings.

dsh Abstracts. Quarterly from Deafness, Speech and Hearing Publications Inc., Gallaudet College, Washington, D.C. Abstracts articles related to hearing, hearing disorders, speech and speech disorders, including foreign journals.

Education Index. From 1932 to the present. Indexes articles from educational periodicals, conference proceedings, and year books.

ERIC (Educational Resources Information Center). Produced by Council for Exceptional Children. More than 589,000 documents on special education materials. Monthly updates.

Hospital Literature Index. From 1945 to present. Indexes studies on administration, planning, and financing of hospitals and related health care institutions.

International Nursing Index. Indexes international nursing journals and nursing articles from non-nursing literature.

Linguistics and Language Behaviors Abstracts. Produced by Sociological Abstracts Inc. More than 72,000 documents on language problems, speech and hearing problems, learning disabilities, and special education. Quarterly updates.

MEDLINE. Produced by NIH-MEDLARS. More than 1,600,000 documents on medicine, including biomedicine, and humanities as they relate to medicine. Monthly updates.

Nursing and Allied Health. Produced by Nursing and Allied Health Literature Corp. More than 46,000 documents. Abstracts from more than 300 journals in nursing and allied health fields. Bimonthly updates.

REHABDATA. Produced by National Rehabilitation Information Center (NARIC). More than 16,000 documents on rehabilitation including commercial publications, government reports, journals, and unpublished documents. Monthly updates.

Research Quarterly, American Alliance for Health, Physical Education and Recreation. Cumulative in 10-year indexes from 1930 to present.

Sport Database. Produced by Sport Information Resource Center. More than 100,000 documents on all aspects of sports, including sports for persons with disabilities. Bimonthly updates.

US Superintendant of Documents, Monthly Catalog of United States Government Publications. 1895 to present. Lists publications issued by all branches of the U.S. government, both the Congressional and the department and bureau publications. Current issues indexed by author, title, subject, and series/report.

Vocational Rehabilitation Index. From 1955 to 1973. Indexes articles from the main vocational rehabilitation journals and government-sponsored reports of vocational rehabilitation projects.

Well-Written Literature Reviews

Amundsen, L. R., DeValhl, J. M., & Ellingham, C. T. (1989). Evaluation of a group exercise program for elderly women. *Physical Therapy, 69*(6), 475–483.

Croce, R., & DePaepe, J. (1989). A critique of therapeutic intervention programming with reference to an alternative approach based on motor learning theory. *Physical and Occupational Therapy in Pediatrics, 9*(3), 5–33.

Hauzlik, J. R. (1989). The effect of intervention on the free-play experience for mothers and their infants with developmental delay and cerebral palsy. *Physical and Occupational Therapy in Pediatrics, 9*(2), 33–51.

Lennox, L., Cermak, S., & Koomar, J. (1988). Praxis and gesture comprehension in 4-, 5-, and 6-year-olds. *American Journal of Occupational Therapy, 42*(2), 99–104.

Longobardi, A. G., Clelland, J. A., Knowles, C. J., & Jackson, J. R. (1989). Effects of auricular transcutaneous electrical nerve stimulation on distal extremity pain: A pilot study. *Physical Therapy, 69*(1), 24–31.

Neuhaus, B. E. (1988). Ethical considerations in clinical reasoning: The impact of technology and cost containment. *American Journal of Occupational Therapy, 42*(5), 288–294.

O'Brien, V., Cermak, S. A., & Murray, E. (1988). The relationship between visual-perceptual motor abilities and clumsiness in children with and without learning disabilities. *American Journal of Occupational Therapy, 42*(6), 359–363.

Stewart, K. B., Brady, D. K., Crowe, T. K., & Naganuma, G. M. (1989). Rett Syndrome: A literature review and survey of parents and therapists. *Physical and Occupational Therapy in Pediatrics, 9*(3), 35–55.

Stratford, P. W., Norman, G. R., & McIntosh, J. M. (1989). Generalizability of grip strength measurements in patients with tennis elbow. *Physical Therapy, 69*(4), 276–281.

Taylor, E. (1988). Anger intervention. *American Journal of Occupational Therapy, 42*(3), 147–155.

Thibodeaux, C. S., & Ludwig, F. M. (1988). Intrinsic motivation in product-oriented and non-product-oriented activities. *American Journal of Occupational Therapy, 42*(3), 169–175.

APPENDIX

C

Sources for Health-Related Statistics

A series of reports are printed by the Public Health Services under the title Public Health Service Publication No. 1000. The most important for therapists are:

Series 3: Analytical Studies. Reports presenting analytical or interpretive studies based on vital and health statistics.

Series 4: Documents and Committee Reports. Final reports of major committees concerned with vital and health statistics.

Series 10: Data from the Health Interview Survey. Statistics on illness, accidental injuries, disability, use of hospital, medical, dental, and other services, and other health-related topics. Based on data collected in a continuing national household interview survey.

Series 11: Data from Health Examination Survey. Data from direct examination, testing, and measurement of national samples of the population provide the basis for two types of reports: (1) estimates of the medically defined prevalence of specific diseases in the United States and the distributions of population with respect to physical, physiological, and psychological characteristics and (2) analysis of relationships among the various measurements without reference to an explicit universe of people.

Series 12: Data from the Institutional Population Surveys. Statistics relating to the health characteristics of people in institutions, and on medical, nursing, and personal care received, based on national samples of establishments providing these services and samples of the residents or patients.

Series 13: Data from Hospital Discharge Survey. Statistics relating to discharged patients in short-stay hospitals, based on sample of patient records in a national survey of hospitals.

Series 14: Data on Health Resources: Manpower and Facilities. Statistics on geographic distribution and characteristics of health resources, including physicians, dentists, nurses, other health manpower occupations, hospitals, nursing homes, outpatient, and other inpatient facilities.

Series 20: Data on Mortality. Statistics on mortality other than as included in annual or monthly reports. Special analyses by cause of death, age, and other demographic variables.

Series 21: Data on Natality, Marriage and Divorce. Statistics on natality, marriage, and divorce other than included in annual and monthly reports. Special analyses by demographic variables; geographic and time series analyses; studies of fertility.

Series 22: Data from the National Natality and Mortality Surveys. Statistics on characteristics of births and deaths not available from the vital records, based on sample surveys, including such topics as mortality by socioeconomic class, medical experience in the last year of life, characteristics of pregnancy, and so forth.

For a list of titles of reports published in these series, write to:
Office of Information
National Center for Health Statistics
Public Health Service, HRA
Rockville, MD 20852

APPENDIX

D

Hardware Resources

Medical Electronics and Equipment News.
Available from:
Reilly Publications Co.
Park Ridge, IL 60068
A semimonthly paper available by subscription. Reports on the availability of instruments including scientific apparatus, electronic devices, laboratory supplies, and material and accessories used in clinical applications, diagnoses, therapy, radiology, surgery, analyses, and research.

Science Guide to Scientific Instruments.
Available from:
Science magazine as an annual supplement.
Lists many instruments and manufacturers.

Directory and Buyer's Guide in Medical Electronics & Equipment News.
Usually in the December issue.
Contains information for equipment for purchases for the upcoming year.

Encyclopedia of Instrumentation and Control. Edited by D.M. Considine, 1971.
Available from:
McGraw-Hill Book Co.
New York, NY 10011
A listing of about 700 entries of instruments and equipment available.

Source of Equipment for Sport Science Laboratories. Edited by R.B. Walker.
Available from:
Canadian Association of Sports Sciences
Guelph, Ontario
Canada

Suppliers of Tests

The Psychological Corporation
757 Third Avenue
New York, NY 10017
One of the largest publishers and suppliers of psychological tests, including aptitude and ability tests, intelligence tests, personality tests, aptitude and interest inventories, reading and vocabulary tests, books on testing.

Stoelting Corporation
1350 South Kostner Avenue
Chicago, IL 60623
Publishers of intelligence tests, form boards, spatial relations tests, coordination tests, motor skill tests, timing and counting devices, biofeedback instruments, sensory-motor apparatus.

J.A. Preston Corporation
60 Page Road
Clifton, NJ 07012
Publishers of sensory-motor equipment, preschool and primary readiness tests, form boards, manual dexterity tests, prevocational skill tests, physical rehabilitation materials, research apparatus and equipment.

Western Psychological Services
12031 Wilshire Boulevard
Los Angeles, CA 90025
Publishers of personality tests, attitudes, traits and leadership inventories, social maturity tests, projective drawing tests, neurological assessments, behavior scales, school readiness tests, special education assessments for learning disabilities, educational achievement tests, perceptual-motor tests, speech and audiometry assessments, health questionnaires, vocational interest and aptitude tests, books on testing, counseling and special education.

Educational and Industrial Testing Service
San Diego, CA 92107
Publishers of personality tests, interest, ability and aptitude inventories, achievement and leadership tests.

Psychological Assessment Resources, Inc.
P.O. Box 98
Odessa, FL 33556
Publishers of achievement and aptitude tests, neuropsychological assessments, personality and intelligence tests.

Institute for Personality and Ability Testing
P.O. Box 188
Champaign, IL 61820
Publishers of personality tests, intelligence tests, and tests of motivation.

APPENDIX

F

Bibliographic Sources for Tests

Buros, O. K. (Ed.). (1978). *The eighth mental measurements yearbook*. Highland Park, NJ: Gryphon Press.
The most comprehensive listing of mental measurement tests. Includes title, author, publisher, and description of most tests in print.

Chun, K. T., Cobb, S., & French, J. R. (1985). *Measures for psychological assessment*. Ann Arbor, MI: Institute for Social Research, University of Michigan.
Title, author, publisher, and description of measures for psychological assessment. A guide to 3,000 original sources and their applications.

Hemphill, B. J. (Ed.). (1982). *The evaluative process in psychiatric occupational therapy*. Thorofare, NJ: Slack Inc.
Describes the psychiatric occupational therapy interview process, projective instruments, observation scales, questionnaires and performance evaluations, and the research methodology used in developing these assessment tools. Each author discusses his or her own instrument.

Robinson, J. P., & Shriver, P. R. (1985). *Measures of social psychological attitudes*. Ann Arbor, MI: Institute for Social Research, University of Michigan.
Title, author, publisher, and description of measures for psychological attitudes.

APPENDIX

G

Principles of the Declaration of Helsinki (World Medical Association)

Adopted by the 18th World Medical Assembly, Helsinki, Finland, 1964, and amended by the 41st World Medical Assembly, Hong Kong, September 1989.

I. Basic Principles

1. Biomedical research involving human subjects must conform to generally accepted scientific principles and should be based on adequately performed laboratory and animal experimentation and on a thorough knowledge of the scientific literature.

2. The design and performance of each experimental procedure involving human subjects should be clearly formulated in an experimental protocol which should be transmitted for consideration, comment and guidance to a specially appointed committee independent of the investigator and the sponsor provided that this independent committee is in conformity with the laws and regulations of the country in which the research experiment is performed.

3. Biomedical research involving human subjects should be conducted only by scientifically qualified persons and under the supervision of a clinically competent medical person. The responsibility for the human subject must always rest with a medically qualified person and never rest on the subject of the research, even though the subject has given his or her consent.

4. Biomedical research involving human subjects cannot legitimately be carried out unless the importance of the objective is in proportion to the inherent risk to the subject.

5. Every biomedical research project involving human subjects should be preceded by careful assessment of predictable risks in comparison with foreseeable benefits to the subject or to others. Concern for the interests of the subject must always prevail over the interests of science and society.

6. The right of the research subject to safeguard his or her integrity must always be respected. Every precaution should be taken to respect the privacy of the subject and to minimize the impact of the study on the subject's physical and mental integrity and on the personality of the subject.

7. Physicians should abstain from engaging in research projects involving human subjects unless they are satisfied that the hazards involved are believed to be predictable. Physicians should cease any investigation if the hazards are found to outweigh the potential benefits.

199

8. In publication of the results of his or her research, the physician is obliged to preserve the accuracy of the results. Reports of experimentation not in accordance with the principles laid down in this Declaration should not be accepted for publication.

9. In any research on human beings, each potential subject must be adequately informed of the aims, methods, anticipated benefits and potential hazards of the study and the discomfort it may entail. He or she should be informed that he or she is at liberty to abstain from participation in the study and that he or she is free to withdraw his or her consent to participation at any time. The physician should then obtain the subject's freely-given informed consent, preferably in writing.

10. When obtaining informed consent for the research project the physician should be particularly cautious if the subject is in a dependent relationship to him or her or may consent under duress. In that case the informed consent should be obtained by a physician who is not engaged in the investigation and who is completely independent of this official relationship.

11. In case of legal incompetence, informed consent should be obtained from the legal guardian in accordance with national legislation. Where physical or mental incapacity makes it impossible to obtain informed consent, or when the subject is a minor, permission from the responsible relative replaces that of the subject in accordance with national legislation.

Whenever the minor child is in fact able to give a consent, the minor's consent must be obtained in addition to the consent of the minor's legal guardian.

12. The research protocol should always contain a statement of the ethical considerations involved and should indicate that the principles enunciated in the present Declaration are complied with.

II. Medical Research Combined with Professional Care (Clinical Research)

1. In the treatment of the sick person, the physician must be free to use a new diagnostic and therapeutic measure, if in his or her judgment it offers hope of saving life, reestablishing health, or alleviating suffering.

2. The potential benefits, hazards and discomfort of a new method should be weighed against the advantages of the best current diagnostic and therapeutic methods.

3. In any medical study, every patient—including those of a control group, if any—should be assured of the best proven diagnostic and therapeutic method.

4. The refusal of the patient to participate in a study must never interfere with the physician-patient relationship.

5. If the physician considers it essential not to obtain informed consent, the specific reasons for this proposal should be stated in the experimental protocol for transmission to the independent committee (I, 2).

6. The physician can combine medical research with professional care, the objective being the acquisition of new medical knowledge, only to the extent that medical research is justified by its potential diagnostic or therapeutic value for the patient.

III. Non-Therapeutic Biomedical Research Involving Human Subjects (Non-clinical Biomedical Research)

1. In the purely scientific application of medical research carried out on a human being, it is the duty of the physician to remain the protector of the life and health of that person on whom biomedical research is being carried out.

2. The subjects should be volunteers—either healthy persons or patients for whom the experimental design is not related to the patient's illness.

3. The investigator or the investigating team should discontinue the research if in his/her or their judgment it may, if continued, be harmful to the individual.

4. In research on man, the interest of science and society should never take precedence over considerations related to the well-being of the subject.

Available from World Medical Association Inc., 28 Avenue Des Alpes, 01210 Ferney-Voltaire, France.

APPENDIX

H

Sample of a Consent Form

ELECTROMECHANICAL TOYS AND EXPLORATION BEHAVIOR IN PROFOUNDLY RETARDED ADULTS

Names of investigators: _____

_____ has been asked to take part in a research study on the effect
(Name of client)
of electromechanical toys on exploration behavior. The purpose of the study is to see if electromechanical toys will encourage clients who have diminished interest in their surroundings to explore and interact with the toy.

_____ will be given a battery-powered toy for fifteen minutes,

three days per week for three weeks, at the _____ State School. His/her behavior will be recorded in writing by a member of the occupational therapy staff to see if his/her exploration behavior changes and if the toy interests him/her. Behavior will be videotape recorded on two separate occasions.

_____ will have the choice to interact with the toy or not.

Participation is entirely voluntary and _____ has the right to withdraw consent and discontinue participation in the study at any time without prejudice to present or

future care at the _____ State School. There is no cost for any part of the study.

No discomfort or risks are anticipated. It is hoped that _____ will enjoy interacting with the toy and may benefit from doing so by learning more about his/her environment. Information from this study will be anonymously coded to ensure confidentiality and

_____ will not be personally identified in any publication containing the results of this study. The videotapes and written material from the study will be kept in a locked cabinet. The videotape recordings will be viewed solely by members of the occupational therapy department and will be destroyed upon completion of data analysis. The parent/ guardian may view any videotape of _____ which is filmed for the study.

_____ OTR, director of the occupational therapy department at the

_____ State School (phone number), will be available to answer any questions you may have concerning the study, the procedures, and any risks or benefits that may arise from participating in the study.

As parent/guardian of the above-named client, I give permission for him/her to participate in the research study described.

A copy of this consent form has been given to me.

Signed _____ Date _____
Parent/Guardian

_____ Date _____
Principal Investigator's Signature

_____ Date _____
Witness Signature

Sample of Permission Form to Use Photographs and Other Media Materials

MEDIA RELEASE

I give permission to the Communications Department of the _____
(Name of facility)

to use materials identifying _____ in the following situations:
(Name of patient/client)

_____ External publications (e.g., professional journals, newspapers, magazines)
_____ Radio programs
_____ Television programs
_____ Internal publications (e.g., facility publications)
_____ Internal/residential building displays (e.g., bulletin boards, photo albums)
_____ Conference materials (e.g., slides, overheads)

_____ Other _____
(specify)

In many cases, the use of the patient's/client's first and last name is not necessary, but can add to the completion of the story or photo. If you do NOT want the last name used, please indicate below:

_____ NO, the use of first and last name is NOT permissible
_____ YES, the first and last names may be used
_____ Only the first name and last initial may be used

I give consent on the condition that the material be used only for the above purpose(s). It is my understanding that I may see the materials before confirming consent or before the material is released. Also, it is my understanding that I will receive verbal notification before any material is used, and that I may place the following restrictions on the material or its use, including time limits:

I give this consent voluntarily, without threat of punishment or promise of special reward. I have been given an opportunity to fully discuss the release and to have my questions answered. I understand that I may withdraw consent at any time prior to release without fear or punishment.

_____   _____
Date   Signature

_____   _____
Date   Signature of parent or guardian

I have fully explained the information above and answered all questions to the best of my ability. It is my opinion that consent has been given knowingly and freely.

_____   _____
Date   Person obtaining consent

                                                 _____
                                                 Title/position

J

Human Subjects Committee Guidelines for Informed Consent from a Children's Hospital

INFORMED CONSENT

One of the most important components of research involving human subjects is that of informed consent.

For the purpose of these guidelines informed consent will be defined as:

Consent freely given by a participant in a research project based upon full disclosure of the procedures that the individual will undergo.

GENERAL INFORMATION

The consent form should be written in terms comprehensible to the layperson and should include all information about the study that any reasonable person would need and want to know. It should, realistically and honestly, express what a participant may expect, and should avoid persuasion by raising false hopes.

Informed consent forms used for research programs are not legal documents, although there have been adverse legal decisions in cases where informed consent was felt to be sufficiently lacking.

Informed consent is to be obtained from every person who agrees to participate in any program falling under the jurisdiction of the Consent Committee. The consent form for each study is to be submitted to the Committee with the approved protocol prior to the beginning of any part of the investigation.

All efforts should be made so that the participant fully understands the information obtained in the informed consent, despite any complicating factors, such as mental incompetence, language difficulties, illiteracy, age, and so forth. If it appears that patients, parents, or guardians are incapable of comprehending this information, the executive officers should be notified and a member of the Consent Committee will be made available. In cases of a language barrier, the executive officer will obtain the assistance of a knowledgeable person in that language to translate the informed consent or interpret during the explanation. Should the participant have questions, and so forth regarding the research once it has begun, the participant will again be provided with an interpreter.

WRITTEN INFORMED CONSENT

A standardized format has been devised in order to facilitate writing of informed consent.

These forms are available from _____. Additional assistance in planning, wording, and developing consent forms may be obtained from

_____.

Using the standardized format, the following elements should be included:

1. Description and explanation of procedure
2. Risks and discomforts
3. Potential benefits
4. Alternatives
5. "Consent"

1. Description and explanation of procedure

The basic procedures of the research should be stated clearly and concisely in non-technical terms. Special note must be made of any part of these procedures that are experimental. The purpose of the study should be described, and the reason this person is being asked to participate should be explained.

2. Risks and discomforts

List in simple terms the most serious risks and those most likely to occur. For each risk or hazard, whenever applicable, answer such questions as: How much will it hurt? How long will it take? What danger will the patient be in? What will be done to counteract adverse effects? Are the side effects reversible? What will be done beforehand to minimize risk or discomfort? Is there inconvenience to the patient regarding time or cost? Could there be psychological harm, invasion of privacy, loss of confidentiality, embarrassment, or social injury?

It is important to state whether risks of experimental procedures or side effects are known.

3. Potential benefits

Potential benefits are considered to be either (1) of direct benefit to the subject or (2) of value to future patients or society as a whole. If it is felt that physical or emotional problems might be uncovered during a study, it might be desirable to state that professional services would be offered to help the problem. If appropriate, results of testing, questionnaires, or interviews might be offered to the child's school or physician if the parent or subject requests it.

4. Alternative

There are sometimes alternative procedures or medications to the ones described, and these should be listed so as to give the subject a clear choice. The risks and benefits of each alternative also should be stated. Where there are no alternatives to a particular treatment, this should be noted. If the only alternative is non-participation, the section can be omitted. This section has to be carefully worded so as not to make a patient feel pressured into participating because the alternatives are made to sound much less desirable.

5. Consent

The following additional items must be contained in every consent form.

1. The assurance that full information regarding the study has been given to the subject.
2. The fact that the physician or investigator is available to answer any inquiries concerning the study.
3. The option of subjects to withdraw from the project at any time without any effect on their treatment or, if hospital employees, their employment.

The following paragraphs are part of the standard format and should be included at the end of the consent document:

I have fully explained to _____

Participant/parent/guardian

the nature and purpose of the above-described procedure and the risks involved in its performance. I have answered and will answer all questions to the best of my ability. I will inform the participant of any changes in the procedure or the risks and benefits if any should occur during or after the course of the study.

_____

Investigator's signature

I have been satisfactorily informed of the above-described procedure with its possible risks and benefits. I give permission for my/my child's participation in this study. I know that

Dr. _____ or his/her associates will be available to answer any questions I may have. If I feel my questions have not been adequately answered, I may request to speak to a member of the Hospital Consent Committee by calling extension

_____. I understand that I am free to withdraw this consent and discontinue participation in this project at any time and it will not affect my child's care. I have been offered a copy of this form.

_____

Signature of participant

_____   _____

Witness signature   Parent/guardian signature

Modification of the wording in these paragraphs may be made in certain cases, depending on the nature of the study.

The parent and/or legal guardian must sign the document, as well as the physician or investigator, and witness. The witness is to the signatures only. In cases where witnesses to the explanation are required, a member of the Consent Committee will fulfill this function.

The consent form containing the original signatures must be placed in the medical record. If there is no medical record — as for volunteers, students, and so forth — then the signed copy must be kept in the investigator's files. A copy of the consent form should always be offered the participant.

If new information occurs during the course of a study, the investigator has the obligation to inform the subject. The consent form should then be revised accordingly and the changes communicated to the executive officer.

B. OTHER TYPES OF CONSENT

1. *Letter.* In some instances, the Committee will approve consents in letter form, particularly when they involve questionnaires or other low-risk studies. These generally occur

in school populations or retrospective studies of former patients when mailings are sent out to individuals not likely to be at the hospital.

2. *Telephone.* At times, the parents of a child to be considered for a study are not available to sign a consent form. In these rare cases, telephone consent can be obtained. The following phrase is added to the consent form:

Since the parents of the child were unavailable, this information has been conveyed to _____ by telephone.

_____
Investigator's signature

_____
Witness to telephone conversation

The investigator should read the consent form to the parent or guardian while a second individual listens to the conversation on another line to witness the fact that consent was given.

3. *Short form.* Occasionally, due to a study's complexity, it is not possible to write a concise consent form. In such instances, the investigator may explain the procedure orally and at length, but present the patients with only a short form to sign. The short form will indicate that all the requirements for informed consent have been met by means of the oral explanation and will include the standard closing paragraphs of written consents. If such form of consent is used, a written summary of what is told the patient should be part of the protocol and must receive Committee approval.

Oral consents should be restricted to extraordinary situations.

C. PARTICIPATION OF CHILDREN IN CONSENT PROCESS

Children should be involved in the consent process whenever appropriate or feasible. They should be as fully informed about the research project as is appropriate for the child's age and should be given the right to refuse participation. It is recommended that a child not be used as a subject in research if there is a conflict between parent and child regarding participation.

It is recommended that children younger than 18 years of age who are capable of understanding a procedure and its ramifications and who agree to participate sign the consent form along with the parent or guardian. This process is left to the discretion of the investigator.

APPENDIX

K

List of Professional Journals and Their Publishers

ADMINISTRATION

Hospital and Health Services Administration; American College of Health Care Executives, Health Administration Press, Ann Arbor, MI

Hospitals; American Hospital Association, American Hospital Publishing Inc., Chicago, IL

Journal of Long-Term Care Administration; American College of Health Care Administrators, Alexandria, VA

Modern Healthcare; Crain Communications Inc., Chicago, IL

Journal of Rehabilitation Administration; Journal of Rehabilitation Administration Inc., Littleton, CO

AGING

Activities, Adaptation and Aging; Haworth Press, Binghampton, NY

Clinical Gerontologist; Haworth Press, Binghampton, NY

Gerontologist; Gerontological Society of America, Washington, DC

Interdisciplinary Topics in Gerontology; Basel, Switzerland (text in English)

International Journal of Aging and Human Development; Baywood Publishing Co. Inc., New York, NY

Journal of Aging and Social Policy; Haworth Press, Binghampton, NY

Journal of Applied Gerontology; Sage Publications Inc., Newbury Park, CA

Journal of Geriatric Psychiatry; Boston Society for Gerontological Psychiatry, Universities Press Inc., Madison, CT

Journal of Gerontology; Gerontological Society of America, Washington, DC

Journal of Women and Aging; Haworth Press, Binghampton, NY

Physical and Occupational Therapy in Geriatrics; Haworth Press, Binghampton, NY

COMPUTER APPLICATIONS

Computers in Human Services; Haworth Press, Binghampton, NY
Computers in Schools; Haworth Press, Binghampton, NY

CRIMINAL JUSTICE

Journal of Offender Counseling, Services and Rehabilitation; Haworth Press, Binghampton, NY
Women and Criminal Justice; Haworth Press, Binghampton, NY

EDUCATION

Special Services in the Schools; Haworth Press, Binghampton, NY

HEALTH CARE

Occupational Therapy in Health Care; Haworth Press, Binghampton, NY
Physical Therapy in Health Care; Haworth Press, Binghampton, NY
Women and Health: The Journal of Women's Health Care; Haworth Press, Binghampton, NY

HOME HEALTH

Home Health Care Series Quarterly; Haworth Press, Binghampton, NY
Journal of Home Health Care Practice; Aspen Publishers Inc., Rockville, MD

HOSPICE

American Journal of Hospice Care; S. DiTullio, 470 Boston Post Road, Weston, MA 02193
Hospice Journal; Haworth Press, Binghampton, NY
Hospice Letter; Health Resources Publishing, Wall Township, NJ

OCCUPATIONAL HEALTH AND VOCATIONAL DEVELOPMENT

Journal of Health and Social Behavior; American Sociological Association, Washington, DC
Journal of Occupational Medicine; American Occupational Medicine Association, Williams & Wilkins, Baltimore, MD

Journal of Occupational Psychology; British Psychological Society, Leicester, England

Journal of Rehabilitation; National Rehabilitation Association, Alexandria, VA

Occupational Health and Safety; Stevens Publishing Corp., Waco, TX

Occupational Health Nurses Journal; American Association of Occupational Health Nurses, Slack Inc., Thorofare, NJ

PHYSICAL MEDICINE AND REHABILITATION

Accent on Living; Cheever Publishing Inc., Bloomington, IL

American Archives of Rehabilitation Therapy; American Association for Rehabilitation Therapy, Little Rock, AR

American Journal of Physical Medicine and Rehabilitation; Williams & Wilkins, Baltimore, MD

American Rehabilitation; Rehabilitation Services Administration, Washington, DC

Archives of Physical Medicine and Rehabilitation; American College of Rehabilitation Medicine, Chicago, IL

British Journal of Occupational Therapy; College of Occupational Therapists Ltd., London, England

Coordinator; J. Berke, Coordinator Publications Inc., Los Angeles, CA

Journal of Rehabilitation; National Rehabilitation Association, Alexandria, VA

Physiotherapy; Chartered Society of Physiotherapy, London, England

Physiotherapy Canada; Canadian Physiotherapy Association, Ontario, Canada

Rehabilitation Counseling Bulletin; American Rehabilitation Counseling Association, Alexandria, VA

Rehabilitation Digest; Canadian Rehabilitation Council for the Disabled, Toronto, Canada

Rehabilitation Education; Pergamon Press Inc., Elmsford, NY

Rehabilitation Literature; National Easter Seals Society, Chicago, IL

Rehabilitation Report; Demos Publications, New York, NY

Sexuality and Disability: A journal devoted to the study of sex in physical and mental illness; Human Sciences Press, New York, NY

PROFESSIONAL ASSOCIATION JOURNALS

American Health Care Association Journal; American Health Care Association, Washington, DC

American Journal of Art Therapy; Vermont College of Norwich University, Montpelier, VT

American Journal of Hand Therapy; American Society of Hand Therapists, Philadelphia, PA

American Journal of Occupational Therapy; American Occupational Therapy Association, Rockville, MD

Journal of Allied Health; American Society of Allied Health Professions, Chicago, IL

Journal of Rehabilitation; National Rehabilitation Association, Alexandria, VA

Occupational Therapy Journal of Research

Physical Therapy; American Physical Therapy Association, Alexandria, VA

Rehabilitation Counseling Bulletin; American Rehabilitation Counseling Association, Alexandria, VA

PSYCHOLOGY AND MENTAL HEALTH

The Clinical Supervisor; Haworth Press, Binghampton, NY

Community Mental Health Journal; Human Sciences Press, New York, NY

Hospital and Community Psychiatry; American Psychiatric Association, Washington, DC

Journal of Family Psychotherapy; Haworth Press, Binghampton, NY

Journal of Organizational and Behavior Management; Haworth Press, Binghampton, NY

Occupational Therapy in Mental Health; Haworth Press, Binghampton, NY

Psychological Medicine: A Journal for Research in Psychiatry and the Allied Sciences; American Psychiatric Association, Cambridge University Press, NY

Prevention in Human Services; Haworth Press, Binghampton, NY

Residential Treatment for Children and Youth; Haworth Press, Binghampton, NY

Schizophrenia Bulletin; National Institute of Mental Health, ADAMHA, Washington, DC

Special Services in the Schools; Haworth Press, Binghampton, NY

APPENDIX

L

Sample Aim and Scope of a Professional Journal

THE OCCUPATIONAL THERAPY JOURNAL OF RESEARCH

AIM AND SCOPE

In 1965, The American Occupational Therapy Foundation, Inc., was chartered as a charitable, scientific, literary, and educational society to "advance the science of occupational therapy . . . and increase the public knowledge and understanding thereof." Toward these ends, the Foundation has provided support for scholarships, publications, and research. Sponsorship of *The Occupational Therapy Journal of Research (OTJR)* is a further expression of the Foundation's commitment to advancing the profession through scientific inquiry.

As its title suggests, the aim of *OTJR* is to provide a dynamic medium for the communication of scholarly writings of potential significance to the field of occupational therapy. The journal seeks to publish original manuscripts pertaining to the impact of activity on the individual, particularly as such activity is applied in a health-related context to prevent disability and to maintain or restore optimal human function or performance.

OTJR will consider submitted manuscripts on a broad scope of subjects of potential concern to occupational therapy researchers. Of particular interest are manuscripts that:

- Demonstrate the value and efficacy of occupational therapy procedures or services.
- Describe new occupational therapy assessment or evaluation approaches or address the standardization, reliability, validity, or innovative application of existing measures.
- Advance the conceptual basis for occupational therapy practice through research that bears on the validity of current theories.
- Propose new theories or paradigms that serve to explain or organize existing data in useful ways.
- Relate to the education of occupational therapy practitioners, particularly as such manuscripts suggest improvements in the educational process on the basis of empirical research.

Additionally, scholarly dialogue is encouraged through letters to the Editor and invited Commentary. Occasionally, the journal will select discussants to critique accepted manuscripts, and such Commentary will be published following designated articles. Readers are welcome to submit thoughtful letters to the editor pertaining to research published in *OTJR*. Other features include Briefs, which present amplified abstracts of completed theses or unpublished research projects; Book, Monograph, and Journal Reviews; and Published Elsewhere, a list of recently published articles of potential interest to occupational therapy researchers.

Full-length manuscripts are evaluated through a blind review process, and selection is based on relevance to the profession, scientific merit, timeliness, and scholarly excellence. All contributors are required to assign exclusive copyright to The American Occupational Therapy Foundation, Inc., and assurance must be given that manuscripts are not under consideration for publication elsewhere. Potential contributors should consult submission guidelines published in the journal under Information for Authors.

APPENDIX

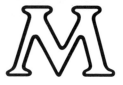

Sample Author's Guides from Professional Journals

SAMPLE 1: PHYSICAL THERAPY: *INSTRUCTIONS TO AUTHORS*

(Reprinted from *Physical Therapy* with the permission of the American Physical Therapy Association.)

MANUSCRIPTS

Physical Therapy, the official journal of the American Physical Therapy Association, represents the science and practice of physical therapy. The Journal is the peer-reviewed (refereed) publication of the Association and, as such, documents the state of the art of physical therapy for the Association and becomes the archives of our professional knowledge.

Purpose of Manuscripts

Manuscripts should contribute to the literature of the profession by providing new information, insights, or ideas. Preference is given to publishing articles that are oriented toward demonstrating clinical implications for the improvement of patient services. Papers regarding basic sciences, education, or administration also are considered.

Manuscripts may be full-length articles or brief reports. (Criteria for acceptable manuscripts of either category may be found in the October 1985 issue of *Physical Therapy* or the APTA *Style Manual*.)

Articles may be reports of research, descriptions of an approach or process, reviews of literature, or presentations of a theory.

Brief reports may be case reports, clinical reports, special communications, or suggestions from the field.

Articles that do not fall in the above categories and that share hands-on advice, undocumented opinions, and new ideas about physical therapy as it relates to direct patient care and clinical management may be submitted to the Association magazine, *Clinical Management in Physical Therapy*.

Preparation of Manuscripts

Before you submit a manuscript, we recommend that you consult the fifth edition of the *Style Manual*, available at $30 per copy from the American Physical Therapy Association (members $20). The manual includes details of acceptable style and format and specifics of manuscript preparation and submission.

Manuscripts that do not follow the APTA guidelines for preparation and submission will not be accepted for review. For examples of acceptable papers, inspect articles in recent issues of *Physical Therapy*. We strongly recommend that you ask your own editorial consultant (and a statistical consultant, if appropriate) to review your manuscript before you submit it to *Physical Therapy*.

For research papers, authors must demonstrate evidence of protection of subjects. The evidence should include statements regarding the use of an informed consent and the approval of the project by a review board or similar body.

When writing, use the active voice to facilitate clarity, succinctness, and preciseness. Avoid terminology that reinforces sex-role stereotyping and questionable attitudes and assumptions about people.

When preparing a manuscript, DOUBLE SPACE every line (including quotations, references, figure legends, and tables). Be sure to include the following:

- *Title page* with the title, the author name(s), and a footnote of biographical data about author(s). (See recent issues of the Journal for specific examples and wording.) Also include notation in footnote if work was supported by a grant or other funding sources or was adapted from a conference presentation.
- *Abstract of 150 words or less.* Research paper abstracts should include purpose, method (e.g., subjects, design, and procedures), results, and conclusion (including clinical implications). Abstracts for other papers should include purpose, summary of key points presented, and statement of conclusion or recommendations. Abstracts are not required for a Suggestion From the Field.
- *Text of 15 pages or less.* Use 1-inch margins, and $8\frac{1}{2}$- by 11-inch bond. State purpose in the introduction. Use appropriate organization and headings such as found in the APTA *Style Manual* or in recent issues. [There follow notes concerning: Manufacturer's information; contributors; references; tables; figures; photographs; appendices.]

Submission of Manuscripts

All manuscripts must be accompanied by transmittal letters containing the following statement:

In compliance with the Copyright Revision Act of 1976, the undersigned author or authors warrant that they have sole ownership of the work submitted, that the work is original and has never been published, and that the author or authors have full powers to grant such rights.

In consideration of the APTA's journal, *Physical Therapy*, taking action in reviewing and editing my (our) submission, the author (authors) undersigned hereby transfer(s), assign(s), or otherwise convey(s) all copyright ownership to the APTA, in the event that such work is published by the APTA in *Physical Therapy*.

In addition, the author or authors hereby grant APTA's journal, *Physical Therapy*, the right to edit, revise, abridge, condense, and translate the foregoing work.

Transmittal letters must be signed by *all* authors of the manuscript. We will send all correspondence to the first author named on the manuscript, unless otherwise instructed.

When submitting a manuscript, include the following:

- Copyright release statement
- One original of the paper
- Four copies of the original paper
- Four originals of each figure

- Permission-to-reprint statements
- Photograph release forms

When submitting a revised manuscript, include the following:

- One original of the revised paper
- Two copies of the revised paper
- Two originals of each revised figure

Send the transmittal letter and the manuscript packet to:
Editor, *Physical Therapy*
American Physical Therapy Association
1111 N. Fairfax Street
Alexandria, VA 22314

Review and Publication

Manuscripts are reviewed and edited to improve the effectiveness of communication between you and the readers and to help you comply with the accepted style of *Physical Therapy*. The identity of the author(s) is kept confidential from all reviewers. (A copy of the Manuscript Evaluation Form used in reviewing manuscripts is available from the APTA.) The entire process from submission to acceptance takes an average of 7.5 months.

Most manuscripts require some revision; both the manuscript and the details of the reviewers' suggestions are sent to the author. If the revisions are not received from the author within three months, the manuscript no longer will be considered for publication, and the original manuscript will be returned to the author.

If your paper is accepted for publication, you will receive a preview of your edited paper to review and approve before it is sent to the printer. When your paper is accepted, you will be asked to provide, if possible, a computer diskette from an IBM or compatible PC, in Word Perfect or ASCII file format. This diskette will expedite the copy editing of your text. About one month before publication, the publisher will invite you to order reprints.

Potential Conflict-of-Interest Statement

Authors are expected to disclose any commercial associations that might pose a conflict of interest in connection with the submitted article. All funding sources supporting the work should be acknowledged in a footnote on the title page. All affiliations with or financial involvement in any organization or entity with a direct financial interest in the subject matter or materials of the research discussed (e.g., employment, consultancies, stock ownership or other equity interest, patent-licensing arrangements) should be cited in a cover letter. This information will be held in confidence by the Editor during the review process. If the manuscript is accepted, the Editor will discuss with the author(s) how best to disclose the relevant information.

Requests for Reprints

Requests for reprints of articles already published should be sent directly to the first author unless otherwise indicated in the biographical data footnote.

Requests for Reproduction

Accepted manuscripts are the property of the Journal. For permission to reproduce an article published in *Physical Therapy*, send request to the Editor.

BOOK REVIEWS AND ABSTRACTS OF CURRENT LITERATURE

[There follows information about applying to be a book reviewer or an abstracter for *Physical Therapy*.]

SAMPLE 2: AUTHOR'S GUIDE FROM THE AMERICAN JOURNAL OF OCCUPATIONAL THERAPY

(Reprinted from the *American Journal of Occupational Therapy* with the permission of the American Occupational Therapy Association.)

The *American Journal of Occupational Therapy* welcomes manuscripts that pertain to occupational therapy. Feature-length manuscripts (12–18 pages) may include (a) reports of research, educational activities, or professional trends; (b) descriptions of new occupational therapy approaches, programs, or services; (c) review papers that survey new information; or (d) theoretical papers that discuss or treat theoretical issues critically. Short manuscripts (3–6 pages) may be (a) descriptions of original therapeutic aids, devices, or techniques; (b) case reports that describe occupational therapy for a specific clinical situation; or (c) opinion essays that discuss timely issues or opinions and are supported by cogent arguments. In addition, the journal publishes letters to the editor and book reviews as space permits and at the discretion of the Editors. All copy is subject to editing. Important considerations are interest to the profession, originality, timeliness, validity, readability, and conciseness.

SUBMISSION

Manuscripts are submitted with the author's explicit assurance that they are not simultaneously under consideration by any other publication. To permit anonymous peer review, send three copies (including three copies of tables, photos, drawings, etc.) to the Editor. In your letter of transmittal, designate the senior author or another person as correspondent. The journal cannot assume responsibility for the loss of manuscripts.

PREPARATION

The entire manuscript, including the abstract, quotations, tables, and references must be typed double-spaced on $8\frac{1}{2} \times 11$ inch white paper, with 1-inch margins.

Title page. Titles should be short and specific and should summarize the main idea of the paper. List three key words or phrases (not mentioned in the title) that highlight important aspects of the material presented in the article. Provide authors' names, degrees, job titles, and current affiliations at the bottom of the page or on a separate sheet. (Include previous work affiliation if the article was written during the time of that affiliation.) Please include city, state, and zip code for workplace, as well as a telephone number where you can be reached.

Abstract. Every feature-length manuscript must have an abstract (maximum of 150 words). The abstract should be factual, succinct, and sufficiently complete to enable the reader to grasp the essence of the paper quickly. An informative type of abstract includes a statement of the problem, method of study, results, and conclusions reached. A descriptive type of abstract indicates the subjects covered, central thesis, sources used, and conclusions.

Text. The introduction should include a statement of purpose (why the manuscript topic is being presented to occupational therapy readers at this time) or an indication of the topic's importance or relevance to the field. The literature reviews should be limited to those citations of primary relevance to the topic and should emphasize the more recent publications.

Acknowledgments. Acknowledgments must be brief. They are typed double-spaced and appear after the text but before the reference page. Acknowledgments to people precede those for grant support. If the article is based on a thesis or on a presentation at a meeting, state this fact following the acknowledgments of people and grants.

References. References must also be typed double-spaced. Follow the style shown in the third edition of the *Publication Manual of the American Psychological Association* (1983), listing references in alphabetical order at the end of the article and providing authors' names and year of publication for in-text citations.

Personal communications or other nonretrievable citations are described in the text. Provide name and date if the information was obtained from a person; provide name, date and address if the information was obtained from an organization. Articles accepted for publication but not yet published can be included as references if you provide the name of the journal or book publisher.

Authors are solely responsible for the accuracy and completeness of the references. You should review and check them thoroughly. See the examples below for commonly used reference listings.

Journal article:
Ottenbacher, K., & York, J. (1984). Strategies for evaluating clinical change: Implications for practice and research. *American Journal of Occupational Therapy, 38*, 647–659.

Book With Individual Author:
Ayres, A. J. (1973). *Sensory integration and learning disorders*. Los Angeles: Western Psychological Services.

Edited Book:
Hopkins, H. L., & Smith, H. D. (Eds.). (1978). *Willard and Spackman's occupational therapy* (5th ed.). Philadelphia: J.B. Lippincott.

Book with Corporate Author and Author as Publisher:
American Psychological Association. (1980). *Diagnostic and statistical manual of mental disorders* (3rd ed.). Washington, DC: Author.

Tables. Tables should be self-explanatory and can be used if they supplement, rather than duplicate, the text. Type tables double-spaced, one on a page. Provide titles for each, and cite them in numerical order in the text.

Figures. Figures can be line drawings, graphs, charts, or photographs. Omit figures that repeat information given in the text or that do not enhance the understanding of the article.

Line drawings, graphs, and charts should be done professionally. Submit photographs as glossy black-and-white prints. Tape photographs onto a white piece of paper and write only on the paper. Do not use paper clips on photographic material. Symbols, abbreviations, and spellings should be consistent with those given in the text. Each figure must be labeled: Specify the figure number and the name of senior author and indicate the figure's orientation (top) with an arrow.

Figures are cited in numerical order in the text. They must have captions, which should be typed double-spaced on a separate sheet of paper and numbered in consecutive order.

A letter of permission to publish (in duplicate) from the subjects must accompany the photographs of all identifiable subjects.

Abbreviations. The use of abbreviations is discouraged. If they are used, they are spelled out on their first appearance.

PATENTS

AOTA's copyright of the *American Journal of Occupational Therapy* only protects articles or works of authors published in the journal from unauthorized copying. It does not protect any items or products mentioned in such articles or works of authors.

Any device, piece of equipment, splint, or other item described with explicit directions for construction in an article submitted to the *American Journal of Occupational Therapy* for publication is not protected by AOTA copyright and can be produced for commercial purposes and patented by others, unless the item was patented, or its patent is pending, at the time the article is submitted.

COPYRIGHT

Authors are required to convey copyright ownership of their manuscripts to AOTA. Manuscripts published in the journal are copyrighted by AOTA and may not be published elsewhere without permission. Permission to reprint journal material for commercial or other purposes must be secured in writing from AOTA's Publications Division.

REVIEW OF MANUSCRIPT

All accepted manuscripts are subject to copyediting. Authors will receive a photocopy of the edited manuscript for review and final approval, as well as reprint order forms. The manuscript must be returned to AOTA by first-class mail within 72 hours. The author(s) assumes final responsibility for the content of the manuscript, including the copyediting.

STYLE/STYLE MANUAL

We have adopted the Publication Manual of the *American Psychological Association* (3rd edition, 1983) as our style guide. Consult the manual for all style questions.

If you have questions about the paper you contemplate submitting, refer to similar papers published in the journal. Alternatively, contact the Editor for writing guidelines regarding the following: Brief or New articles, Case Reports, Program Descriptions, Scientific Papers, Review Papers, and Procedures on Special Issues.

APPENDIX

N

Sample Timetables from Students' Theses

SAMPLE 1

This timetable is based on the fall semester 1989 and the 15-week spring semester 1990.

1. Pilot study conducted and any necessary amendments made to the rating scale.	Fall semester, 1989
2. Pre-test on students using the Leadership Skills and Responsibilities Rating Scale.	Second week of Spring semester. January 22, 1990
3. Students will co-lead ILS groups.	Weeks 3–13 February–April, 1990
4. Results of pre-test tabulated.	Week 3. Feb. 5, 1990
5. Post-test students using the rating scale.	Week 12. April 2, 1990
6. Results of post-test tabulated.	Week 13. April 9, 1990
7. Results and Discussion sections written.	Weeks 14–16. April–May, 1990
8. Chapter 1 written	November 1989
9. Chapter 2 written	September 1989–January 1990
10. References and Appendices written	January 1990
11. Meet with readers	Every 4 weeks

SAMPLE 2

Sequence of Procedures and Time Frame

1. Pilot study to evaluate appropriateness of questions	2 weeks
2. Revise survey	1 week
3. Printing of survey and cover letter	1 week
4. Obtain list of pediatric occupational therapists in Massachusetts	2 weeks
5. Address, stamp, and stuff envelopes	1 week
6. Response time	3 weeks
7. Send follow-up post cards	1 week
8. Response time	2 weeks
9. Tabulate and evaluate data	2 weeks
10. Analysis of data	1 week
11. Write up results and discussion	4 weeks
	Total 20 weeks
On-going review of literature	Weeks 1–16

SAMPLE 3

Timetable

October–November 1988	Thesis proposal to committee
December 1988	Approval of human subjects committee
November 1988–January 1989	Review of the literature
December 1988–February 1989	Data collection and analysis
February 1989–March 1989	Write up results
March 1989	Final draft to readers
May 1989	Ready for hearing

SAMPLE 4

The proposed time frame for this study is as follows:

January	Proposal hearing
January, February	Human subjects committees review (2)
February–April	Data collection and analysis
May, June	Results and discussion

SAMPLE 5

Timetable

Late December to mid-January — Complete thesis proposal
Mid-January to early February — Thesis proposal hearing
February — Human subjects committee review
February to mid-April — Collect data and work on literature review
End April to end May — Complete data analysis
June to August — Complete writing of thesis
September — Thesis hearing
End September — Make revisions

INDEX

An "f" following a page number indicates a figure.

a priori method, 99
abbreviations, 219
abstracts, 17–19, 170, 171, 190–191, 218
activity dimension, 94
affective meaning, 94
affective factors, 95
American Journal of Occupational Therapy, 18,
    166, 167, 171, 218–220
American Medical Association Stylebook/Editorial
    Manual, 167
American Physical Therapy Association Style
    Manual, 167, 170, 173, 215
American Psychological Association Style Manual.
    See Publication Manual of the American
    Psychological Association
analysis of covariance (ANCOVA), 120, 121, 128
analysis of variance (ANOVA), 120, 121, 127–128,
    129
anonymity, 138
appendices, 176
articles, as records, 96
artifacts, as records, 96
assumptions, 76–78, 81, 96–97, 175
audiotapes, 63, 203–204
  as records, 96
author's guide, 167, 172, 215–220
Author's Guide to Journals in Psychology,
    Psychiatry, and Social Work, 167
Author's Guide to Journals in Sociology and
    Related Fields, 167
Author's Guide to Journals in the Health Field, 167
average score, 121

background of the study, 29–30, 174
bar graph, 151 example, 152*f*, 153*f*
behavioral research, 139
bias, 41, 42, 61, 102, 137, 146
bimodal scores, 122
bipolar scale, 94
BMDP—Biomedical Data Package, 129
books, as records, 96
Books in Print, 17
boundaries, 74–81
British Books in Print, 17
British Journal of Occupational Therapy, 166–167
British Journal of Physiotherapy, 166

Canadian Journal of Occupational Therapy, 166
card catalog, 16–17
case conferences, 96
case study, 1, 46, 61–63, 96, 98–101, 140
causal inferences, 100

cause-and-effect relationship, 46, 60, 126
central tendency, 122, 146, 147
charts, 148, 151, 153, 170, 219
chi-square, 120, 121, 123, 124, 170
classic experimental design, 52–53, 123
closed-ended question, 93–94, 99
clothing, as records, 96
coding, 99, 148
cohort designs, 57–58
computer searching, 18, 19–20, 24
computers, use of, 101, 118–119, 129, 176
concept coding, 99
conceptual framework, 78–79, 81
conclusions, 154–156
confidentiality, 137, 175
consent form, 137, 138, 201–202, 203–204
content analysis, 101
continuous data, 120
control, 40–41, 42, 43, 44, 45, 46, 52, 54, 57, 58, 59,
    102, 119, 121, 123, 124, 175
  the subject as own control, 45*f*
control period, 44, 45
convenience samples, 55–57, 169
copyright, 167, 172, 173, 219, 220
correlated groups t test, 124
correlation coefficient, 60, 126
correlation tests, 126–127
correlational research, 8, 45–46, 60, 147, 175
cover letter, 93, 139
cross-section. 60, 61
Current Index to Journals in Education (CIJE), 18

data, 60–61
  categories, 119–121
data analysis, 60, 63, 98–102, 118–130, 137, 140,
    175
data bases, 19–20
data collection, 61, 63, 64, 66, 90–98, 130, 137, 140,
    141, 169, 175, 176
  sample sheet, 56*f*
Declaration of Helsinki, 199–200
deductive reasoning, 1
definition of terms, 74–76, 175
degrees of freedom, 170
delimiting factor, 79
dependent variable, 40, 43, 44, 46, 52, 54, 58, 59,
    99, 119, 123, 127, 128, 175
descriptive research, 45, 126
descriptive statistics, 119, 121–122, 149, 150
descriptors, 19
diaries, as records, 96
discrete data, 120
Dissertation Abstracts, 19